ESSENTIALS OF ENDOSCOPIC SINUS SURGERY

Essentials of Endoscopic Sinus Surgery

Heinz Stammberger, M.D.
Professor and Head
Department of General ENT–Head and Neck Surgery
University of Graz Medical School
Graz, Austria

Michael Hawke, M.D.
Professor of Otolaryngology and Pathology
University of Toronto
Toronto, Canada

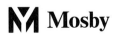 Mosby

St. Louis Baltimore Boston Chicago London Madrid
Philadelphia Sydney Toronto

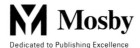

Publisher: George Stamathis
Editor: Robert Hurley
Associate Developmental Editor: Karyn Fell Taeyaerts
Project Manager: Nancy C. Baker
Project Supervisor: Deborah Thorp
Proofroom Manager: Barbara M. Kelly
Designer: Nancy C. Baker
Manufacturing Supervisor: Betty Richmond

Copyright © 1993 by Mosby–Year Book, Inc.

Printed in the United States of America

Composition by Graphic World
Printing/binding by Walsworth

Mosby–Year Book, Inc.
11830 Westline Industrial Drive
St. Louis, Missouri 63146

Library of Congress Cataloging in Publication Data
Stammberger, Heinz.
    Essentials of functional endoscopic sinus surgery/Heinz
Stammberger, Michael Hawke.
      p.   cm.
    Includes bibliographical references and index.
    ISBN 1-55664-386-1
    1. Paranasal sinuses—Endoscopic surgery.   I. Hawke, Michael,
M.D.   II. Title.
    [DNLM: 1. Paranasal Sinuses—surgery.   2. Endoscopy.   WV 340
S783ea 1993]
RF421.S78 1993
617.5'23—dc20
DNLM/DLC
for Library of Congress   93-4631
                                                   CIP

1 2 3 4 5 6 7 8 9 0 GW/CD/WA 97 96 95 94 93

This work is dedicated to
Professor Doctor Walter Messerklinger,
Scholar and Physician,
and to
Doctor Karl Storz,
Instrument maker
The work in this book is a classic example of the benefits of a close partnership between a pioneering physician and a creative instrument maker.

Contributors

Lalitha Shankar, M.D.
Department of Radiology
St. Joseph's Hospital
Toronto, Canada
Assistant Professor of Radiology
Faculty of Medicine
University of Toronto
Toronto, Canada

Kathryn Evans, M.D.
Consultant Otolaryngologist
Gloucester, United Kingdom

Preface

This text, *Essentials of Functional Endoscopic Sinus Surgery,* was conceived by Brian Decker and the authors as a basic, practical, and readily affordable introductory text that would provide the reader with the "essential" information about the Messerklinger technique and the concepts of functional endoscopic sinus surgery. This introductory textbook has its origins in Heinz Stammberger's classic textbook, *Functional Endoscopic Sinus Surgery: The Messerklinger Technique,* published in 1991 by B.C. Decker, Philadelphia. It is hoped that the affordability of this text will enable our knowledge and experience to reach the widest possible audience.

Nasal endoscopes have opened up a new world for the otorhinolaryngologist, and as a result of Professor Messerklinger's work, nasal endoscopy has become an irreplaceable, routine procedure without which modern functional surgery would not be possible. In combination with modern imaging techniques, particularly computerized tomography, nasal endoscopic examination provides diagnostic possibilities unimagined a few decades ago. The brilliance and color of the photographs in this text demonstrate the excellent cooperation and support provided by the Karl Storz Company and by its owner and developer Doctor Karl Storz.

It must always be remembered that accurate diagnosis and, when possible, treatment by medical means are the hallmarks of functional endoscopic sinus techniques. When endoscopic surgical intervention is indicated, the surgeon must remember that the guiding concept is the preservation of structure and the re-establishment of function by preserving the mucous membranes. This is accomplished by removing as little as possible and preserving as much of both the bony structures and their covering mucous membranes as possible. The result is a "tailor made" operation designed for the individual patient's specific needs.

The Messerklinger technique of functional endoscopic sinus surgery that was developed in Graz has rendered largely obsolete those major radical procedures directed towards the connecting paranasal sinuses. The Messerklinger technique changed operations on the frontal sinus into an operation on the frontal recess, and operations on the maxillary sinus into a procedure on the ethmoidal infundibulum and/or on the clefts of the lateral nasal wall.

The endoscope is also of great help in the local and medical therapy of infectious processes of the paranasal sinuses. Target-oriented, focused therapy of the middle meatus practically negates the use of surgical intervention, when in the past fenestration of the inferior meatus would have been almost routine.

Under endoscopic guidance, a total sphenoethmoidectomy *can* be performed, when necessary. The great advantage of the Messerklinger technique, however, is that such a procedure can be largely avoided. To put it bluntly, the endoscope is the instrument that helps us *to avoid* surgery.

Heinz Stammberger, M.D.
Michael Hawke, M.D.

Acknowledgments

We wish to thank Brian Decker for conceiving this work, Gino Hasler for his fantastic art, and Doctor Lalitha Shankar and Doctor Kathryn Evans for providing Chapter 3, "Imaging of the Paranasal Sinuses." The continuous and invaluable support that we both have received from the Karl Storz company and in particular from Dr. Karl Storz, Mrs. Sybill Storz-Reling, and Mr. Hans Joachim Lunemann are gratefully acknowledged. Finally, and most importantly, we wish to thank our wives, Doloris and Naneve, for their patience and forbearance during the work on this book and its predecessor.

Heinz Stammberger, M.D.
Michael Hawke, M.D.

Contents

1 Basic Principles of Functional Endoscopic Sinus Surgery

MUCOCILIARY CLEARANCE: MECHANISM FOR SECRETION TRANSPORTATION

The health and normal function of the paranasal sinuses and their lining mucous membranes depends primarily on two important factors: ventilation and drainage. Normal ventilation of the sinuses requires both a patent sinus ostium and a patent pathway (prechamber) connecting the ostium to the nasal cavity. Normal drainage of the sinuses is a complex function of both the production of mucus (mucus secretion) and the ciliary mechanisms that transport the mucus through and out of the sinus and into the nasal cavity (the mucociliary transportation mechanism). Normal drainage of mucus from the sinuses depends to a large extent on the amount of mucus produced, its composition, the effectiveness of the ciliary beat, mucosal resorption, and the condition of the ostia and the ethmoidal clefts or prechambers into which the respective sinus ostia open.

An unimpeded flow of air during inspiration through the nose is also important in the transportation of mucus, because forced inspiration creates suction, or negative pressure, which promotes the transportation of mucus out of the sinuses.

NORMAL PATHWAYS OF MUCOCILIARY CLEARANCE

Our knowledge of the pathways along which the cilia transport mucus is largely the result of the work of Messerklinger, who followed the animal experiments of Hilding Sr. Messerklinger's studies were based on the observation that human nasal and paranasal sinus mucosa and their ciliary activity survive the death of the individual for 24 to 48 hours. Although the cilia beat somewhat slower after death, they retain exactly the same pattern and pathways as they did in life.

In his original studies, Messerklinger used fresh cadaver heads, staining the mucus by adding dust particles or different types of powders. He was able to study the pathways of mucus transportation in all of the paranasal sinuses by taking time-lapse movies. Simultaneously during sinus operations, Messerklinger expanded on these observations using sterile dermatol powder to learn more about the effects of disease on the mucociliary transportation mechanism.

These studies were done primarily with the operating microscope in the 1950s and the early 1960s. It was the need to further investigate both the normal and the abnormal pathophysiology of the mucociliary transportation patterns in patients without traumatic or invasive techniques that led Messerklinger to search for a better tool for this purpose. He ultimately selected the nasal endoscopes as his primary investigative instruments. Today, with powerful cold light endoscopes, the ciliary transportation mechanism can be easily studied, because almost all of the mucosal surfaces can be directly visualized. Not only can the effect of ciliary action and secretion transport be observed, but the actual ciliary beat becomes easily visible in the light-reflecting areas of the mucosa.

After experimentation with a variety of stains and particles, we have found that the patient's own blood provides the best substance to color the secretions. Either the few drops of blood that flow into the maxillary sinus when a trocar is inserted can be used, or in some cases a few drops of the patient's blood can be taken from a vein and instilled into the floor of the sinus through the trocar sleeve. Usually after 2 or 3 minutes, depending on the prevailing mucosal pathologic condition, this blood-tinged mucus can be followed on its way toward the ostium as illustrated in Fig 1–1. Sometimes it may be necessary to add a little heparin or citrate to the blood to prevent coagulation.

One of Messerklinger's most important discoveries was the observation that the mucus produced in the sinuses does not travel in a random fashion to their respective ostia but follows definite pathways that appear to be genetically determined. Although these pathways may be impeded or even blocked by various pathologic conditions, their direction is not significantly altered.

MUCUS TRANSPORTATION PATHWAYS IN MAXILLARY SINUS

In the maxillary sinus, secretion transportation starts from the floor of the sinus in a stellate pattern. The mucus is then transported along the anterior, medial, posterior, and lateral walls of the sinuses and along the roof. All of these secretion routes converge at the natural ostium of the maxillary sinus (see Fig 1–1). When the mucus has passed through the natural ostium of the maxillary sinus it has not yet reached the free middle meatus, and next it must pass through a very narrow and complicated system of clefts in the lateral nasal wall.

The natural ostium of the maxillary sinus normally opens into the floor of the posterior third of the ethmoidal infundibulum, which is bordered by the uncinate process medially and the papyraceous lamina of the orbit laterally (see Chapter 2). The ethmoidal infundibulum opens into the middle meatus through the hiatus semilunaris (a two-dimensional cleft bordered by the anteroinferior face of the ethmoidal bulla posteriorly and the posterior free margin of the uncinate process anteriorly). The mucus from the maxillary sinus is transported via the infundibulum through the hiatus semilunaris. After leaving the hiatus semilunaris, the mucus is then transported over the medial face of the inferior turbinate posteriorly into the nasopharynx (see Fig 1–1).

Not all areas of the maxillary sinus mucosa seem to transport mucus uniformly, and from time to time the endoscopist can see one area of the mucosa transporting mucus faster than its neighboring areas, with the mucus overtaking the other secretions on their way to the ostium. After a few minutes the slower areas may speed up as the faster area slows down. This phenomenon of "secretion expressways" can be found both in cases of abnormal secretion

A

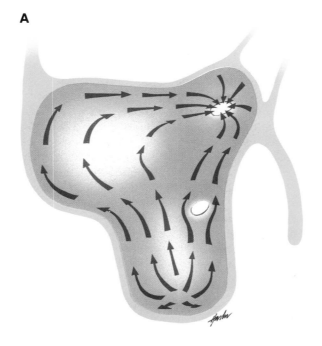

B

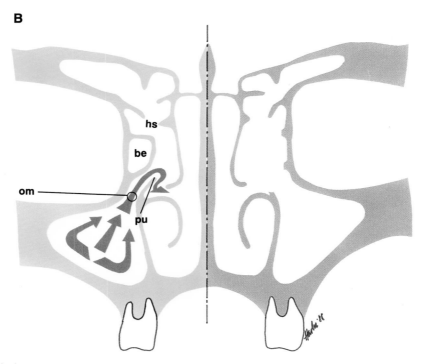

FIG 1–1.
Schematics of the normal transportation pathways of mucus inside **(A)** and moving out of **(B)** maxillary sinus. *be* = bulla ethmoidalis, *hs* = hiatus semilunaris, *om* = maxillary ostium, *pu* = uncinate process. (After W. Messerklinger.)

and in apparently normal sinuses. We do not know whether this phenomenon is an artifact caused by the light and warmth of the endoscope or by the trauma of its insertion or whether it serves a special purpose, such as to avoid the jamming up of mucus at the narrow ostial passage.

Secretions from the maxillary sinus are always transported via the natural ostium, even when one or more accessory ostia are present in the area of the nasal fontanelles and even in those patients in whom a patent window in the inferior meatus has been surgically created (inferior meatal antrostomy). This is one reason why we no longer perform inferior meatal antrostomies. Although an inferior meatal nasoantral window may provide ventilation for a diseased maxillary sinus and thus help to normalize conditions in the sinus, an inferior meatal window cannot achieve sufficient active outwardly directed transportation of mucus.

Accessory ostia are frequently present in the fontanelles of the maxillary sinus. These accessory ostia are usually bypassed by the normal secretion pathways. In cases of higher viscosity, the entire mucous layer may move over such an accessory ostium without any mucus leaving the sinus.

MUCUS TRANSPORTATION PATHWAY IN FRONTAL SINUS

The frontal sinus is the only sinus in which there is active *inwardly directed* transportation of mucus. Mucus is transported into the frontal sinus along the interfrontal septum, then laterally along its roof, and back medially via the floor and the inferior portions of the posterior and anterior walls of the sinus. The mucus then exits the frontal sinus ostium via the lateral side of its ostium. Not all of this mucus leaves the sinus after one "round trip." This is the result of a whorl-like formation in the ciliary pattern, which may be present in a shallow sulcus immediately above the frontal ostium as well as inferior to it in the frontal recess. A variable amount of the mucus leaving the sinus comes into contact with the inwardly directed transport route, and thus may recycle through the sinus several times (Fig 1–2).

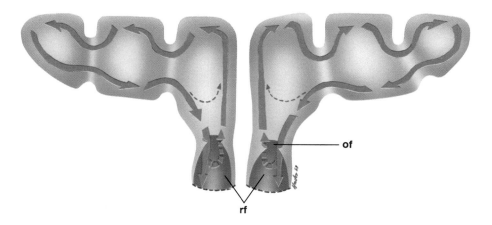

FIG 1–2.
Schematic of secretion transport inside and out of frontal sinus. *of* = frontal sinus ostium, *rf* = frontal recess.

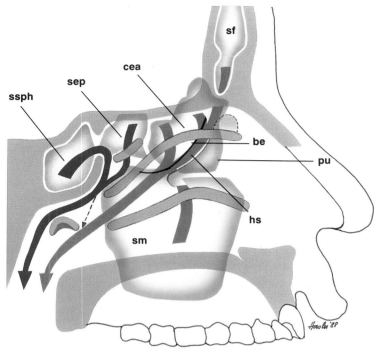

FIG 1–3.
Schematic of normal secretion transport pathways in lateral nasal wall. *be* = ethmoidal bulla, *cea* = anterior ethmoidal complex, *hs* = hiatus semilunaris, *pu* = uncinate process, *sep* = posterior ethmoidal sinus, *sf* = frontal sinus, *sm* = maxillary sinus, *ssph* = sphenoidal sinus.

Once it has passed out of the frontal sinus ostium, the mucus is transported through a narrow cleft of variable dimensions, the frontal recess. This recess drains either directly into the ethmoidal infundibulum from above or medially to the ethmoidal infundibulum when the infundibulum ends with a superior blind pouch. The frontal recess, depending on anatomic variations, may also collect secretions from other ethmoidal compartments, including secretions from the lateral sinus, from the agger nasi, from a pneumatized middle turbinate, and from the most anterior ethmoidal cells. In addition, the mucous transportation routes from the superior aspect of the head of the middle turbinate and from the front of the middle meatus may also connect with the transport routes out of, and even more important into, the frontal sinus. Eventually the secretions from the frontal sinus merge with the secretions from the maxillary sinus, and together they are transported back into the nasopharynx (Fig 1–3).

MUCOUS TRANSPORTATION PATHWAYS FROM ANTERIOR AND POSTERIOR ETHMOIDAL AND SPHENOIDAL SINUSES

If the ostium of an ethmoidal air cell is located in its floor, its mucus is usually transported directly toward the ostium. If, however, the ostium is located higher in one of the walls (e.g., in the posterior wall of the bulla ethmoidalis), there is usually a spiral transportation pattern directed toward the ostium.

The border between the anterior and posterior ethmoidal sinuses is the ground lamella of the middle turbinate (see Chapter 2). All cells opening anteroinferiorly to the ground lamella are anterior ethmoid cells, and drain into the middle meatus. All air cells that open posteriorly and superiorly to the ground lamella are posterior ethmoid cells, and drain via the superior meatus into the sphenoethmoidal recess (see Fig 1–3). When there is a supreme, or fourth, turbinate with cells in the supreme meatus, these cells also drain into the sphenoethmoidal recess.

In the sphenoidal sinus, depending on the location of the ostium, there usually is spiral transportation of mucus toward the ostium, passing subsequently into the sphenoethmoidal recess.

MUCUS TRANSPORTATION PATHWAYS ALONG LATERAL NASAL WALL

Two major routes of mucociliary transportation can usually be identified in the lateral nasal wall (see Fig 1–3). The first route combines the secretions from the frontal and maxillary sinuses and the anterior ethmoidal complex. The secretions from these sinuses usually join in or near the ethmoidal infundibulum, and from there are transported over the free rear margin of the uncinate process and along the medial surface of the inferior turbinate toward the nasopharynx. At this point the secretions pass anteriorly and inferiorly to the eustachian tube orifice. Active transportation continues up to the borderline of the ciliated and the squamous epithelium in the nasopharynx. From this point the secretions are moved by gravity, and are assisted ultimately by the swallowing mechanism.

The second major route combines the secretions from the posterior ethmoidal cells and from the sphenoidal sinus. The secretions from these two sinuses join in the sphenoethmoidal recess, and then are transported toward the nasopharynx posteriorly and superiorly to the eustachian tube orifice. Occasionally minor amounts of secretion from the superior meatus near the posterior end of the middle turbinate may join the first or inferior secretion pathway. The eustachian tube is thus situated like a breakwater between these two secretion pathways. The secretions from the nasal septum are transported more or less vertically downward to the floor of the nose and then backward, where in most cases they join the first secretion pathway to pass anteriorly and inferiorly to the eustachian tube.

EFFECTS OF DISEASE ON MUCUS TRANSPORTATION

The normal transportation of mucus from the sinuses can be adversely affected by various disease processes. The amount and nature of the mucus produced may be altered, and ventilation and drainage from the sinus ostia may also be affected by the disease process.

If the composition of the mucus is altered so that the mucus produced becomes more viscous, the rate of transport toward the ostium will slow considerably and the gel layer become demonstrably thicker. In such cases, the viscous secretion can reach the ostium, even though it is apparently too thick to pass through the ostium. This results in a collection of thick mucus at the ostia, which finally slips back down to the floor as it succumbs to the effects of gravity. Depending on the prevailing conditions, this thick mucus may be dissolved and then transported away or its cycle back toward the ostium may be repeated and the secretion retained in the sinus for a variable period.

When there is a lack of mucus secretion or if a loss of humidity at the mucosal surface cannot be compensated for by the glands and the goblet cells, the mucus becomes more viscous and the sol phase may become extremely thin, allowing the gel phase to come into constant contact with the cilia, thereby impeding their action.

In cases of bacterial or viral superinfection, not only may the mucosal glands be infected, but the entire mucosal surface may be partially destroyed or paralyzed and thus unable to carry out its mucociliary clearance function. A variety of ciliary or mucosal dysfunctions or malfunctions, such as immotile cilia syndrome, cystic fibrosis, and allergic rhinitis, can also severely impair mucociliary clearance.

If pathologic changes occur in the nasal or paranasal sinus mucosa and the nature or quantity of the mucus is altered (e.g., the purulent or highly viscous thickened secretions found in acute or chronic sinusitis) or if the composition of the mucus becomes more viscous, the normal secretion transport routes may undergo significant changes.

KEY ROLE OF ETHMOIDAL PRECHAMBERS IN VENTILATION AND DRAINAGE OF FRONTAL AND MAXILLARY SINUSES: PRIME CONCEPT OF FUNCTIONAL ENDOSCOPIC SINUS SURGERY

The two largest and clinically most important sinuses, the frontal and maxillary sinuses, both communicate with the middle meatus via very narrow and delicate clefts, or *prechambers*. The frontal sinus ostium opens into a funnel-shaped cleft, the frontal recess, which in textbooks is usually referred to as the nasofrontal duct. On a sagittal section, the floor of the frontal sinus and the frontal recess have an hourglass configuration, the narrowest point of which is the frontal sinus ostium (see Chapter 2). We believe the term "frontonasal duct" to be a misnomer, because usually no tubular structure corresponding to an actual "duct" can be identified. The maxillary sinus ostium opens into a cleft in the lateral nasal wall, the ethmoidal infundibulum.

Both of these clefts, or prechambers, are part of the anterior ethmoid and fulfill an important role in the ventilation and drainage of these sinuses. The mucosal surfaces in these prechambers are closely approximated, and in such narrow clefts the mucus, especially when more viscous or otherwise patholog-ically altered, can more easily be transported away and thus the sinus more efficiently drained because the ciliary beat can work in these narrow areas on the mucous layer from two or more sides. Similarly, in an ostium the cilia can act on the mucus in a circular fashion.

If, however, in these clefts the opposing mucosal surfaces come into intense contact and are firmly pressed against each other as the result of mucosal swelling, this pressure may seriously interfere with the drainage and ventilation of the larger dependent sinuses because the ciliary beat is immobilized and consequently the mucus is no longer transported away. When the area of contact is extensive, the ciliary beat may stop completely. The active transpor-tation of mucus can then continue only peripheral to these areas of intense contact.

Despite the fact that initially these areas of contact are clinically almost invisible, small areas such as these may be the underlying cause of severe problems. They can irritate nasal function, disturb the nasal cycle, and cause reactive hypersecretion of the surrounding mucosa, as well as cause sinus headaches or recurring infections of the larger dependent sinuses. If mucosal swelling and mucus retention occurs in one of the key areas (prechambers) such as the infundibulum or the frontal recess, ventilation and drainage of the dependent larger sinus may become impaired and the secretions of that sinus retained. When the area of blockage becomes larger or infection develops, the retained mucus provides an ideal nutrient for both viral and bacterial growth, thus creating a vicious cycle. Allergens and other noxious substances may adhere longer at these contact areas, possibly promoting sensitization.

Because of poor ventilation, the pH of the involved sinus will fall, and this decrease in pH will in turn slow ciliary movement and cause mucus of a higher viscosity to be produced. Because of the blockage of the prechamber and the ciliary insufficiency, these secretions may not be able to leave the sinus for a considerable period, if at all. The hypoxia and the accumulated retained mucus provide ideal conditions for the growth of pathogens. Infection and toxins may additionally impair mucosal function, setting up a vicious cycle.

The clinical symptoms in such cases will be those of "typical" maxillary or frontal sinusitis. The underlying cause of the infection, however, will be found in one of the ethmoidal prechambers and not in the diseased major sinuses themselves (Fig 1–4)! If these ethmoidal prechambers are considerably diseased, the subordinate, or dependent, larger sinuses simply cannot help but become secondarily involved (i.e., infected), because their ventilation and drainage are compromised.

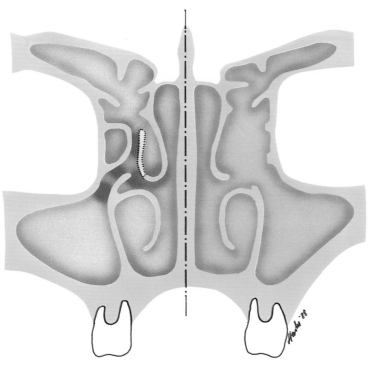

FIG 1–4.
Schematic of diseased ethmoidal sinus **(left)** and after functional endoscopic sinus surgery **(right)**.

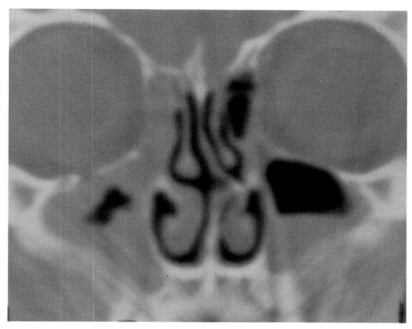

FIG 1–5.
CT scan of bilateral infundibular disease with secondary maxillary sinusitis. See text for discussion.

Any abnormality, whether infection, allergy, trauma, tumor, or anatomic variation, that blocks the entrance into the middle meatus, the hiatus semilunaris, or the infundibulum itself or narrows these already very narrow systems of clefts may predispose to or promote partial or complete blockage of the maxillary or frontal sinus ostia. Depending on the individual circumstances (e.g., if superinfection occurs), not only may this give rise to continuing problems such as nasal obstruction, headache, or postnasal discharge, but these abnormalities may also be responsible for recurring episodes of acute or chronic frontal or maxillary sinusitis.

This concept is clearly demonstrated by computed tomography (CT), as shown in Figure 1–5. Pronounced disease of the anterior ethmoidal sinus is present on the right side, completely blocking the ethmoidal infundibulum and causing marked thickening of the mucosa lining the maxillary sinus. Anterior ethmoidal disease need not necessarily be so severe, as can be seen on the other side in Figure 1–5, where a relatively small but critically located lesion situated exactly in the infundibulum has blocked the infundibulum, causing an air-fluid level in the left maxillary sinus.

Such changes are visible only by tomography or CT scan, and the plain sinus radiographs in this patient who had recurring bilateral episodes of acute maxillary sinusitis demonstrated only a massive opacification, suggesting an air-fluid level in the maxillary sinuses during the acute phase of the disease, but not the underlying causes in the ethmoid complex. This case reinforces the fact that plain sinus radiographs are inadequate for identification of the underlying causes of chronic recurring sinusitis.

SPREAD OF INFECTION INTO FRONTAL AND MAXILLARY SINUSES

In the frontal sinus, mucus is actively transported into the sinus along the interfrontal septum on both sides (see Fig 1–2). Apart from being inhaled into the sinuses, pathogens are deposited by the airflow at the entrance to the middle meatus, where they adhere to the mucous blanket. Because of the confluence of the secretion pathways from the entrance to the middle meatus with the pathways of the infundibulum and the frontal recess, these pathogens may be transported into the frontal sinus, where conditions are ideal for growth. If the self-healing capacity of the sinus mucosa or medical treatment is insufficient to clear the sinus, acute or chronic recurring frontal sinusitis will develop.

The mechanism by which pathogens may enter the maxillary sinus can be studied during maxillary sinoscopy. Thick viscous mucus can frequently be seen entering the maxillary sinus through accessory ostia in one or both of the nasal fontanelles. Once this mucus enters the maxillary sinus, it is transported upward along the natural pathways inside the sinus toward the maxillary sinus ostium, from which it exits the sinus.

In some cases these thick secretions can reenter the maxillary sinus through an accessory ostium, and the mucus may continue to circulate in an endless circle. As long as the natural ostium is patent, this finding may not be of special significance. If, however, the natural maxillary ostium is blocked by disease or when nasal infection is present, this inwardly directed route of transportation through an accessory ostium is one way by which pathogens may be transported into the maxillary sinus from the nose. If the natural ostium is blocked, these infected secretions cannot leave the sinus, and maxillary sinusitis may result.

Sometimes during sinoscopy it is almost impossible to identify the natural ostium of the maxillary sinus, especially when the mucosa is swollen. However, if the patient performs a Valsalva maneuver (pinching the nose and blowing against the closed nostrils), air usually bubbles into the maxillary sinus through its ostium, thereby indicating its position. In many cases, when the patient attempts to blow the nose harder, infected secretions may be forced back into the maxillary sinus from the ethmoidal prechambers.

MESSERKLINGER CONCEPT OF FUNCTIONAL ENDOSCOPIC SINUS SURGERY

The Messerklinger concept for endoscopic diagnosis and treatment of inflammatory diseases of the nose and the paranasal sinuses is based on the clinical observation that most infections of the larger sinuses are rhinogenic. In other words, it usually is the disease within the nose that spreads into the paranasal sinuses. Despite the fact that the clinically dominant symptoms may result from the diseased frontal or maxillary sinus, in most cases the underlying causes are not to be found in the infected sinuses but in the clefts of the lateral wall of the nose.

The function and patency of these normally narrow clefts of the anterior ethmoidal sinus are key to the health of the larger paranasal sinuses. These clefts act as prechambers to the maxillary and frontal sinuses, providing ventilation and drainage for these larger sinuses. Many anatomic variants can narrow these prechambers even more and thereby predispose to recurrent sinus infections (see Fig 1–4).

An exact diagnostic evaluation of the condition of the lateral nasal wall comprised of a diagnostic endoscopic nasal examination and tomography is a prerequisite for the Messerklinger technique.

Messerklinger's surgical concepts were developed from his endoscopic findings, with the goal of treating the diseased areas in the ethmoidal prechambers rather than at the secondarily involved larger sinuses. He observed that when medical treatment was unsuccessful, an accurate and usually limited surgical clearing of the key diseased ethmoidal areas performed under endoscopic guidance frequently was successful in curing the diseased and secondarily involved larger sinuses. As a result, radical surgical procedures on the frontal and maxillary sinuses can usually be avoided.

SUMMARY

Drainage and ventilation of the larger sinuses is essential to the maintenance of their normal function. The ventilation and drainage pathways of the maxillary and frontal sinuses pass from their ostia through very narrow and complicated clefts, or prechambers, before they reach the free middle meatus. These clefts, the ethmoidal infundibulum and the frontal recess, respectively, are parts of the anterior ethmoidal sinus. The frontal and maxillary sinuses are therefore *dependent sinuses* whose health and normal function are subordinate to the health and function of their prechambers in the ethmoidal sinus and lateral nasal wall.

Those disorders that produce any additional stenosis of these already very narrow key areas may result in the contact of opposing mucosal areas with mucus retention, and if they become infected, smaller or larger areas of subacutely or chronically diseased mucosa may persist.

These stenotic areas may be clinically free of symptoms until the nasal cavity becomes infected. If the infection spreads into these key areas and produces complete or partial obstruction of the prechambers or of the ostia of the larger dependent sinuses, the clinical symptoms of acute or chronic infection of the maxillary or frontal sinus will follow. Despite the fact that the symptoms of infection in these larger sinuses are usually the clinically dominant symptoms, the actual underlying cause is generally not to be found in the larger sinuses themselves but in the clefts of the anterior ethmoidal sinus in the lateral nasal wall.

As a result, most of the inflammatory diseases of the frontal and maxillary sinuses are *secondary diseases* (i.e., rhinogenic), caused by infection within the nasal cavity and the anterior ethmoidal sinus. In more than 90% of our patients, the underlying cause of the infection in the frontal and maxillary sinuses can be identified as a lesion in the ethmoidal sinuses located in the lateral nasal wall.

These were the most significant conclusions about the causes and pathophysiology of sinusitis that resulted from Messerklinger's endoscopic studies of the early 1950s and 1960s. Messerklinger also observed that after limited resection of disease and clearing of the key areas in the anterior ethmoidal sinus, with reestablishment of drainage and ventilation via the natural pathways, even massive mucosal pathologic conditions in the dependent frontal and maxillary sinuses usually healed without these sinuses having been directly touched themselves. Mucosal changes, which up to that time had been regarded as "irreversible," returned to normal in a few weeks after what were usually minimal endoscopic procedures.

CONCLUSIONS

1. The frontal and maxillary sinuses are subordinate to the anterior ethmoid. They are ventilated, and their mucus is drained into the nose via the anterior ethmoidal sinus. Their physiologic and pathologic condition therefore depends on the health of the anterior ethmoid.

2. Infections of the frontal and maxillary sinuses are usually rhinogenic, spreading from the nose through the compartments of the anterior ethmoidal sinus to the frontal and maxillary sinuses.

3. When sinus infection does not resolve or recurs constantly, a focus of infection usually persists in one of the narrow clefts of the anterior ethmoidal sinuses. These foci interfere with normal nasal function, and from these areas infection may spread locally to involve the prechambers and the larger sinuses.

4. This is true even for many infections that were originally dentogenic, traumatic, or bloodborne in which the sinusitis keeps recurring after the primary source of infection has been cured.

5. The narrow or stenotic areas primarily involved are the ethmoidal infundibulum at the entrance to the maxillary sinus and the frontal recess at the entrance to the frontal sinus.

6. After the clearing of disease in the clefts of the anterior ethmoidal sinus and the reestablishment of ventilation and drainage via the physiologic routes, even massive changes in the dependent sinuses usually heal without their having been touched.

2 Endoscopic Anatomy of Lateral Nasal Wall and Ethmoidal Sinuses

For radical surgery of the past, a precise definition of the clefts of the ethmoid was of limited significance, because during these procedures more or less all components of the ethmoid system were removed and the maxillary, frontal, and ethmoidal sinuses all were opened wide. Only with the introduction of endoscopic diagnosis and microsurgery did precise description and definition of these clefts become critical. The following description of the anatomy of the lateral nasal wall and ethmoidal sinuses presents concepts and a nomenclature based on the developmental history of this area, which has proved satisfactory for endoscopic diagnosis and therapy over several decades.

ETHMOID BONE

The ethmoid bone consists of a paired bony scaffolding held together by a horizontally oriented plate, the lamina cribrosa (cribriform plate), the name of which is derived from its multiple perforations, which serve as conduits for the olfactory filaments (Fig 2–1). In the midline, separating the two laminae cribrosae, there is anteriorly a superiorly pointing spur, the crista galli. Inferiorly, in the midline opposite the crista, lies the perpendicular plate of the ethmoid bone.

The initially confusing bony structure (appropriately named the "ethmoid labyrinth") that is attached to the lamina cribrosa makes up the bulk of the ethmoid bone. With some imagination it can be likened to a box of matches standing on end. It is subdivided internally by bony septa and has the following characteristics.

The system has its own bony margins in only two directions. Laterally, the lamina papyracea forms a thin bony division from the orbit. In some persons this lamina may have dehiscences (in which case, the periosteum of the ethmoid bone and that of the orbit lie adjacent to each other). Such dehiscences provide a pathway through which an inflammatory process in the ethmoidal sinus can spread into the orbit. Medially, toward the nasal cavity, the ethmoid is bordered by the middle turbinate (first ethmoid turbinate) and by the superior turbinate (second ethmoid turbinate). Occasionally there may be an uppermost supreme turbinate (third ethmoid turbinate).

The ethmoidal bone is open in all other directions. It can be approached anteriorly through the middle, superior, and when present, supreme meatus.

FIG 2–1.
Schematic drawing of the ethmoid
and frontal bones. *1* = crista galli;
2 = lamina cribrosa; *3* = septum
nasi; *4* = lamina lateralis of lamina
cribrosa; *5* = fossa olfactoria
between 1, 2, and 4; *6* = lamina
papyracea; *7* = concha media;
8 = concha superior; *9* =
ethmoidal clefts and cells, open
superiorly; *10* = os frontale with
foveolae ethmoidales.

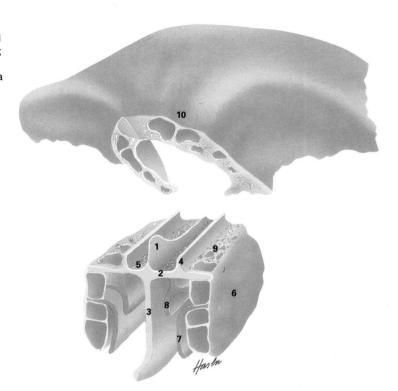

Posteriorly and inferiorly, the ethmoid clefts open into the corresponding nasal passages and finally into the choanae. A part of the posterior cells of the posterior ethmoid borders the sphenoidal sinus. This means that the anterior surface of the sphenoid constitutes the major component of the posterior wall of the posterior ethmoidal cells, which have no bony wall of their own, even here.

That the ethmoid bone is *open cranially* (see Fig 2–1) is extremely important. These open cells and clefts are effectively closed by appropriate downward extensions of the frontal bone that form the roof of the ethmoid. The frontal bone extends with its ethmoidal foveolae across the top of the ethmoidal cells and clefts. The bony base of the roof of the ethmoid is thus provided primarily by the frontal bone. This is of great significance in the behavior of fractures, the development of cerebrospinal fluid (CSF) fistulas, and the possibility of iatrogenic injuries (see Chapter 11). The most anterior and superior clefts of the ethmoid assume in most people a funnel shape because of the "superposition" of the frontal bone. The ethmoid can be intelligently described and understood only in relation to the bony, connective tissue and mucous membrane structures in its immediate, topographic vicinity.

BONY STRUCTURES OF LATERAL NASAL WALL

The bony formations arising from the medial aspect of the ethmoid, known as the turbinates, are really the ends of bony lamellae that traverse the entire ethmoid. They extend laterally to the lamina papyracea, superiorly to the lamina cribrosa, and between the ethmoidal foveolae to the frontal bone. If an attempt is made to reduce the ethmoidal labyrinth in an adult to the identifiable *ground*

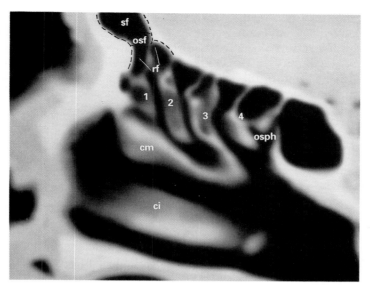

FIG 2–2.
This sagittal CT scan of a cadaver demonstrates the ground lamellae persisting in an adult. Note the hourglass-like contour of the floor of the frontal sinus, which narrows toward the frontal sinus ostium and widens again in the frontal recess *(dotted lines)*. *1* = uncinate process; *2* = ethmoidal bulla; *3* = ground lamella of the middle turbinate; *4* = ground lamella of the superior turbinate; *sf* = sinus frontalis; *osf* = ostium sinus frontalis; *osph* = ostium sinus sphenoidalis; *cm* = concha media; *ci* = concha inferior (the maxilloturbinal).

lamellae, the following picture emerges (Fig 2–2). The first, incompletely developed lamella is represented by the uncinate process. The second ground lamella is the bulla lamella. The intact bulla lamella extends to the base of the skull and separates the frontal recess from the more posteriorly located segments of the anterior ethmoid. If an intact, closed bulla lamella extends far anteriorly, the frontal recess becomes very narrow. This bulla lamella clearly has a decisive influence on the shape of the frontal recess. Pneumatization of the bulla lamella results in the formation of the ethmoidal bulla. The third ground lamella, corresponding to that of the middle turbinate, is the most constant and completely formed lamella and separates the anterior and posterior ethmoidal labyrinths. The fourth ground lamella is formed by the superior turbinate. The occasionally present, smaller supreme turbinate is a fifth lamella. The passages between these ground lamellae are designated the interturbinal meatus.

Further subdivision of the ethmoidal labyrinth results from the formation of more or less developed transverse septa in the interturbinal meatus. Occasionally there are only small, incomplete ridges, but there may also be bony septa that divide the interturbinal meatus almost completely and form cells and cavities that communicate with the interturbinal meatus only through a small ostium. Development of these transverse septa explains why occasionally the ethmoidal infundibulum (as a remnant of the interturbinal meatus) may be further subdivided. In its most anterior part, this can lead to the development of recesses, as seen clearly in the anatomic specimen in Figure 2–16. Initially these recesses are small, but may become larger, and are referred to as "cells." These "infundibular cells" complicate the anatomy, particularly in the passage from the uppermost part of the infundibulum to the frontal recess.

All of this makes it clear that the number of cells in both the anterior and posterior ethmoid labyrinths depends on the development of the septa in the interturbinal meatus. In rare cases, if there are no septa at all, the ethmoidal labyrinth may consist of a single cell that corresponds to the original configuration of the interturbinal meatus.

Variations, disturbances, and anomalies in the formation of the ground lamellae and in the septation of the interturbinal meatus explain not only the variability in the number of cells in the anterior and posterior ethmoidal sinuses but also the variable ratio of the volume of these two areas. As emphasized in the discussion of the ground lamella of the middle turbinate, the border between the anterior and posterior ethmoidal sinuses may become severely obscured by invaginations of the cells. Posterior ethmoidal cells can displace the ground lamella far anteriorly and make it appear to lie within the anterior ethmoidal sinus. In contrast, anterior ethmoidal cells may, in extreme cases, extend to the anterior wall of the sphenoidal sinus.

As Zuckerkandl (1882), Hajek (1916), and Killian (1896) have stated, the only certain point of reference for the topographic orientation of an ethmoidal cell is its ostium. Those cells that open into the middle meatus belong to the anterior ethmoidal labyrinth; those that open into the superior meatus belong to the posterior ethmoidal labyrinth. The ground lamella is the border between the anterior and posterior ethmoidal labyrinths.

Uncinate Process

When looking from the medial side at the lateral nasal wall of an anatomic preparation in which the vertical portion of the middle turbinate has been resected, one can see two distinct bony structures: the uncinate process and the ethmoidal bulla (Fig 2–3).

The uncinate process is a thin, almost sagittally oriented bony leaflet that runs in a sickle-shaped curve from its anterosuperior end posteroinferiorly. If one ignores the numerous fine bony spicules at its posterior end and at its anteroinferior border, the uncinate process resembles a slightly bent hook or a boomerang. Its posterior margin is sharp, concave, and lies roughly parallel to the anterior surface of the ethmoid bulla, located just behind it. The fine bony spicules at the posterior end of the uncinate process attach to the lamina perpendicularis of the palatine bone and inferiorly to the corresponding ethmoidal process of the inferior turbinate. (The inferior turbinate is a bony structure, separate from the ethmoid.) The ascending, anterior convex margin of the uncinate process is in contact with the bony lateral nasal wall, and can extend as far as the lacrimal bone. The uppermost segment of the uncinate process is hidden by the insertion of the middle turbinate. This upper segment of the uncinate process runs a variable course. It can extend to the base of the skull or it may turn laterally (either partially or completely) and insert into the lamina papyracea (see Fig 2–15). It may also turn frontally and fuse with the insertion of the middle turbinate. There may be further divisions, inlet formation, or combinations of all of these. A more detailed description of these variations is found in the discussion of the ethmoidal infundibulum.

In the bony skeleton, there are almost always defects between the uncinate process and the inferior turbinate that are covered with dense connective tissue, which is a continuation of the periosteum, and by the mucous membranes. These defects in the bony skeleton, which open into the maxillary sinus, should not be confused with its natural ostium. These are the structures that Zuckerkandl called the anterior and the posterior nasal fontanelles. Because these fontanelles do not have a bony base, this portion of the lateral nasal wall is known as the *membranous area*. The anterior nasal fontanelles lie anterior to the inferior insertion of the uncinate process, whereas the posterior nasal fontanelles are located posterior to the posteroinferior attachment of the uncinate process.

The concave, free posterior margin of the uncinate process usually does not fuse with any other bony structure. Between the posterior free margin and the anterior surface of the ethmoidal bulla is a sickle-shaped cleft, frequently only 1 to 2 mm wide, which Zuckerkandl called the hiatus semilunaris. Through the hiatus semilunaris, a path leads anteriorly into a three-dimensional space, lateral to the uncinate process, called the ethmoidal infundibulum.

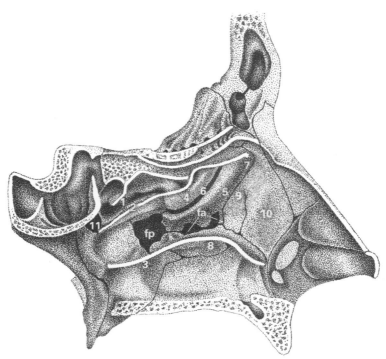

FIG 2–3.
Bony structures of the lateral nasal wall. *1* = edge of resected superior turbinate; *2* = edge of resected middle turbinate; *3* = edge of resected inferior turbinate; *4* = ethmoidal bulla; *5* = uncinate process; *6* = hiatus semilunaris between the ethmoidal bulla and the uncinate process; *7* = agger nasi; *8* = inferior turbinate bone; *9* = lacrimal bone; *10* = processus frontalis of the maxilla; *11* = sphenopalatine foramen; *fa* = anterior (inferior) nasal fontanelle; *fp* = posterior nasal fontanelle.

Ethmoidal Bulla and Lateral Sinus

The ethmoidal bulla is the most constant and usually the largest cell of the anterior ethmoid. It sits like a bleb, medial to the lamina papyracea, and is created by the pneumatization of the bulla lamella. Occasionally an ethmoidal bulla is poorly developed, and may even be totally absent. In the series of ethmoids operated on by us, the incidence of minimal or absent pneumatization of the ethmoidal bulla is 8%.

When extensively pneumatized, the ethmoidal bulla can fill the middle meatus like a balloon. Posteriorly the ethmoidal bulla may fuse with the ground lamella of the middle turbinate over a variable distance. Superiorly the bulla lamella can reach the roof of the ethmoid sinus as a frontally oriented plate, thus forming the posterior wall of the frontal recess. This division may be vestigial or completely absent, in which case there is a direct communication between the frontal recess and a pneumatized space located above the bulla, the sinus lateralis, or lateral sinus of Grünwald. Depending on its size, a lateral sinus can be bounded inferiorly by the roof of the ethmoidal bulla, laterally by the lamina papyracea, superiorly by the roof of the ethmoid sinus, and medially by the middle turbinate. Dorsally a lateral sinus can extend far posteriorly and inferiorly between the ethmoidal bulla and the ground lamella of the middle turbinate. This cleftlike extension can appear sickle shaped when approached from anteromedially, and was called by Grünwald the superior hiatus semilunaris.

Ground Lamella of Middle Turbinate

The most anterior superior insertion of the middle turbinate is adjacent to the ethmoid crest of the maxilla, where it produces an anterior bulge called the agger nasi. The posterior end of the middle turbinate is attached to the ethmoid crest of the perpendicular process of the palatine bone.

The intervening area of insertion of the middle turbinate into the lateral nasal wall can be divided into three parts (Fig 2–4). As can be clearly seen from its medial side, the anterior third of the middle turbinate is entirely vertical and inserts directly into the base of the skull at the lateral edge of the lamina cribrosa. From here the line of insertion turns laterally and reaches the lamina papyracea, where it proceeds sharply inferiorly. When it is viewed from the

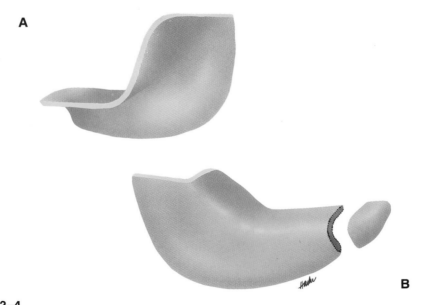

FIG 2–4.
Schematic drawing of the ground lamella of the right middle turbinate. **A,** as seen laterally and anteriorly. **B,** as seen medially and posteriorly. The tip of the posterior turbinate end is shown cut off to demonstrate both the vertical and horizontal parts of the middle turbinate in the posterior third of the middle meatus. For details, see text.

medial side, we can see only the free, vertical segment of the middle turbinate in this middle area. The bony plate of the ground lamella, which is located almost entirely in the frontal plane and consists of the insertion of the middle turbinate on the lamina papyracea, can be seen only after adequate dissection. In the last third of its insertion, the ground lamella of the middle turbinate takes a usually easily identifiable sharp turn toward the horizontal. This horizontal part of the ground lamella forms the roof of the posterior third of the middle meatus. The free, medial, vertical part of the turbinate gradually tapers up to the posterior end of the turbinate.

We can thus distinguish three sections of the insertion of the middle turbinate, which lie in different planes:

1. The anterior third of the middle turbinate inserts vertically in a purely sagittal direction on the lateral end of the lamina cribrosa, directly across from the lamina lateralis.
2. In its middle third, the middle turbinate is attached to the lamina papyracea by its vertically running frontally oriented ground lamella.
3. In its posterior third, the now almost horizontal ground lamella forms the roof of the posterior third of the middle meatus and is fixed to the lamina papyracea or to the medial wall of the maxillary sinus.

This serpentine insertion along different planes—vertical, frontal, and horizontal—contributes significantly to the stability of the middle turbinate. It is therefore not surprising that after resection of the posterior two thirds of the middle turbinate, as recommended by several surgical schools, the remainder of the anterior segment becomes unstable. Even in endoscopic surgical procedures, when manipulations are required in the posterior ethmoidal or sphenoidal sinuses, perforations through the frontal portion of the ground lamella should not be so large that the stability of the middle turbinate is compromised.

The middle section of the ground lamella is worthy of special mention because this frontally oriented attachment plate does not necessarily present a smooth or uniform surface. Well-pneumatized anterior ethmoidal cells can cause this plate to bulge posteriorly, giving it a posterosuperior orientation. This is especially common when a lateral sinus is fully developed. Occasionally such extensively developed anterior ethmoidal cells may extend almost to the sphenoidal sinus. Conversely, the posterior ethmoidal cells can cause the middle section of the ground lamella of the middle turbinate to bulge anteriorly. Occasionally the superior nasal meatus can develop anteroinferiorly to such extent that either it makes the ground lamella of the middle turbinate bulge forward or, in some cases, the superior nasal meatus extends into the bony lamella of the middle turbinate, producing a concha bullosa of the middle turbinate (described by Grünwald as an interlamellar cell).

Because of its numerous variations, the appearance of the ground lamella may be extremely variable, which may make its identification intraoperatively, or even radiologically extremely difficult (see Chapter 8).

Posterior Ethmoidal Sinus

The ground lamella of the middle turbinate is the dividing line between the anterior and posterior ethmoidal sinuses. All cells and clefts belonging to the posterior ethmoidal sinus open posteriorly and above the ground lamella in the superior (and occasionally in the supreme) meatus.

The volume of the posterior ethmoidal sinus depends largely on the structure and the course of the ground lamella of the middle turbinate. The number of cells in the posterior ethmoidal sinus depends primarily on whether the ground lamella of the superior (and the supreme) turbinate extends to the lamina papyracea and on whether there are further subseptations present. The number of cells and clefts that make up the posterior ethmoidal sinus varies between one and five.

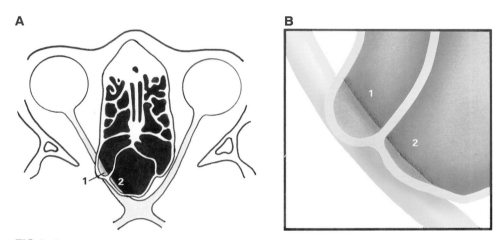

FIG 2–5.
A, schematic drawing showing the relationship of the optic nerve to the lateral wall of a posterior ethmoidal cell (Onodi cell, or sphenoethmoidal cell) and the sphenoid sinus. Note how far lateral to the anterior sphenoid sinus wall the Onodi cells may pneumatize. **B,** detailed view. *1* = optic nerve bulging into an Onodi cell; *2* = optic nerve bulging into the sphenoid sinus.

The behavior of the most posterior cells of the posterior ethmoidal sinus, however, is of the greatest importance to the surgeon, because these posterior cells can develop laterally along, and even superiorly over, the sphenoidal sinus. Such extensive development can extend so far that the most posterior point of a posterior ethmoidal cell can extend laterally 1.5 cm beyond the anterior wall of the sphenoidal sinus. The sphenoidal sinus may also be bypassed to the same extent superiorly by the posterior ethmoidal cells. These cells, named Onodi cells after their Hungarian descriptor, can come into an intimate spatial relationship to the optic nerve (Fig 2–5). The optic nerve may appear prominently on the lateral wall of an Onodi cell, and may in fact be surrounded by these cells. The internal carotid artery may also impinge into the lateral wall of the posterior ethmoidal cells (Fig 2–6).

Under no circumstances should a surgeon assume that the anterior wall of the sphenoidal sinus is always directly behind the most posterior point of the last posterior ethmoidal cell. In the presence of an Onodi cell, the anterior wall of the sphenoid sinus does not run frontally, but in an occasionally very acute angle from *anteromedial to posterolateral.*

A

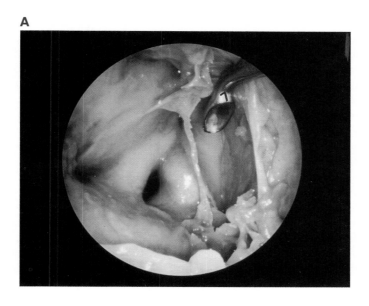

B

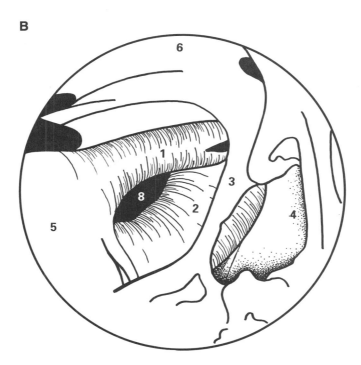

FIG 2–6.
A, an Onodi cell in a right posterior ethmoidal sinus. Note the typically triangular or pyramid-shaped appearance with the tip of the pyramid pointing dorsolaterally. 0-degree lens, cadaveric dissection.)
B, schematic representation. *1* = optic nerve; *2* = carotid artery bulging into the posterior ethmoidal and sphenoid sinuses; *3* = resection line of the anterior wall of the sphenoid sinus; *4* = mucosa of the sphenoid sinus moved medially; *5* = lamina papyracea in the vicinity of the apex of the orbit; *6* = roof of the posterior ethmoidal sinus; *7* = spoon entering the sphenoid sinus; *8* = pneumatized recess between 1 and 2.

If during a surgical procedure it becomes necessary to open the anterior wall of the sphenoidal sinus by way of the anterior and posterior ethmoids, it is highly advisable to stay *as far medial and inferior as possible.* After perforation of the ground lamella, one must never make the mistake of dissecting posterolaterally along the lamina papyracea to seek the sphenoidal sinus behind the last fringes of the Onodi cells. *This is the precise spot where the optic nerve is most likely to be injured.*

In endoscopic procedures, the Onodi cells frequently appear as pyramidal outgrowths of the posterior ethmoidal sinus in a posterolateral or superior direction, with the tip of the pyramid pointing posteriorly away from the surgeon. This is best seen with the 0-degree lens (see Fig 2–6).

The lamina papyracea that forms the lateral wall of the posterior ethmoid is very thin in this area and may show dehiscences, through which the orbital contents may prolapse into the posterior ethmoid (see Chapter 11). Because of the small number of cells in the posterior ethmoidal sinus, the lamina papyracea can usually be seen over a considerable extent during an endoscopic procedure, and in some cases yellow orbital fat can be identified shining through the lamina papyracea. In continuation of a prominent apex of the orbit, the bulge of the optic nerve can be seen on the lateral wall of the posterior ethmoid sinus.

Sphenoidal Sinus

The degree of pneumatization of the sphenoidal sinus may vary considerably, even in the adult. If the cavities are symmetric in the body of the sphenoidal sinus, they are usually divided sagittally by a septum almost exactly in the midline. In some cases pneumatization of the sphenoidal sinus may be so extensive that it involves not only the entire sinus but also the clivus down to the foramen magnum, and may extend laterally all the way to the foramen lacerum. Anteriorly the pneumatization may extend into the septum, and anteriorly and laterally may involve the root of the pterygoid process. It is not uncommon for an extensively pneumatized sphenoidal sinus to be separated from the maxillary sinus by only a thin bony wall.

In cases of extensive pneumatization the maxillary nerve (V_2) may bulge into the lateral wall of the sphenoidal sinus, and in extreme cases may be entirely surrounded by pneumatization. The canal of the vidian nerve may also bulge into this area from the floor of the sphenoidal sinus. There is generally an inverse relationship between the extent of pneumatization and the thickness of the wall of the sphenoidal sinus. The more extensive the pneumatization the thinner the walls.

The ostia of the sphenoidal sinus are usually located in the sphenoethmoidal recess, medial to the superior or supreme turbinate, where they can usually be well seen with an endoscope. The shape of the sphenoidal sinus ostia varies widely; they may be slitlike, oval, or round, and there may be two or more ostia on one side. Occasionally it is possible to examine the interior of the sinus itself through a wide natural ostium.

The floor of the sphenoidal sinus is occasionally composed of ridges, covering the vidian nerve. The medial and superior walls are usually smooth, and the superior wall may balloon out from pressure of the sella turcica (hypophysis).

Two bulges in the lateral wall of the sphenoidal sinus are of critical clinical significance. These are the bulges produced by the optic nerve and the carotid artery. Depending on the degree of pneumatization, these two bulges may be barely noticeable or obvious (Fig 2–7). If the anterior clinoid process is also pneumatized, there may be a deep recess between the optic nerve and the internal carotid artery, pointing laterally and superiorly between the optic nerve and the internal carotid artery.

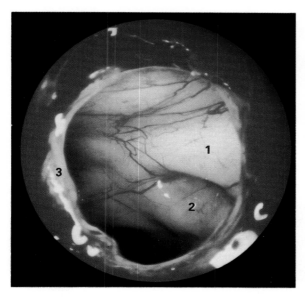

FIG 2–7
Endoscopic view of a normal left sphenoid sinus. (0-degree lens.)
1 = optic nerve; *2* = internal carotid artery; *3* = margin of perforation in the anterior sphenoid wall.

The more superior bulge of the optic nerve extends from the front toward the back, and usually disappears gradually toward the posterior wall. Occasionally the optic nerve runs along an arcuate course medially toward the optic chiasm, which then can be seen bulging into the lumen of the sphenoidal sinus. The internal carotid artery lies adjacent to the sphenoidal sinus during its passage through the cavernous sinus, producing a variable bulge in the lateral wall of the sphenoidal sinus (see Figs 2–7 and 2–8). In extreme cases this bulge may be very prominent, and the bulges of both carotid arteries may almost make contact in the midline. We have confirmed Kennedy's findings and found that in almost 25% of all anatomic preparations that we examined the bony canal covering the internal carotid artery was partially dehiscent. In several cases the artery was entirely uncovered (except by the periosteum and the mucosa of the sphenoidal sinus) over an area 10 by 6 mm. A dehiscence of the bony wall covering the optic nerve was present in a smaller percentage of cases, and in only about 6% was the bone over the optic nerve "clinically dehiscent." By this we mean that the bone provided no resistance to a carefully probing instrument, which could be pushed in easily and could have led to an injury to the optic nerve.

The direction of the septa that can be found in the sphenoidal sinus is also of clinical importance. It is not unusual to find additional septa alongside the median septum, and occasionally two to three complete subseptations may be encountered. Occasionally the single septum may lie in an asymmetric position, dividing the sinus into one large and one small cavity. The course of the septum is not always median, and it frequently deviates laterally and superiorly in its posterior course and inserts into the bony bulge over the optic nerve or the internal carotid artery. Awareness of this is particularly important if the septa in the sphenoidal sinus are scheduled to be perforated or removed.

A

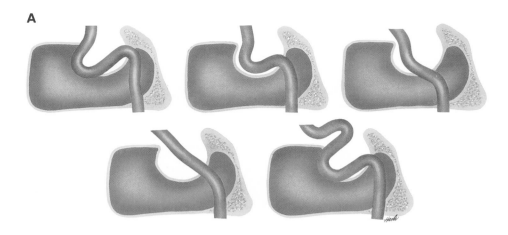

B

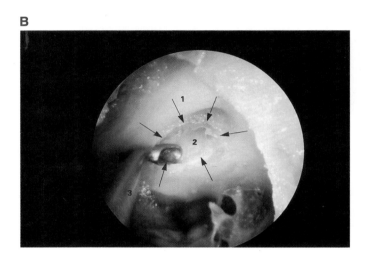

FIG 2–8.
A, schematic drawing showing variations in the course of the internal carotid artery in relation to the sphenoid sinus. The stretched versions are more likely to be encountered in younger individuals. These variations may result in different patterns of bulges of the internal carotid artery in the walls of the sphenoid sinus. **B,** a view into a left sphenoid sinus (cadaveric dissection). (0-degree lens.) *1* = optic nerve; *2* = bulge of the internal carotid artery with bone dehiscence in an area 8 by 5 mm *(arrows)*; *3* = spoon (J-curette) palpating dehiscent carotid for demonstration.

As mentioned, particular attention must be paid during a surgical procedure to the relationship of the sphenoidal sinus to the cells of the posterior ethmoid. The most posterior point of an Onodi cell of the posterior ethmoid may extend up to 1.5 cm beyond the most anterior point of the anterior wall of the sphenoidal sinus. This is especially important if the sphenoidal sinus is to be opened endoscopically via the ethmoid. The anterior wall of the sphenoidal sinus must never be sought behind the furthermost, "deepest" point of the posterior ethmoid, because this is the precise point where the risk of injury to the optic nerve is the greatest (see Figs 2–5 and 2–6).

ROOF OF ETHMOID BONE AND ANTERIOR ETHMOIDAL ARTERY

Because the ethmoid bone is open superiorly, at least over its anterior two thirds, the "roof" for these open cells and ethmoidal clefts is provided by the frontal bone. The frontal bone covers these open spaces with its foveolae ethmoidales. In this area the frontal bone is both thicker and denser than the adjacent bony ethmoidal structures. This difference is greatest medially, in the transition from the thick bony lamellae of the frontal bone to the much thinner lamellae of the ethmoid. This occurs where the frontal bone abuts against the primarily vertical lateral lamella of the lamina cribrosa (see Fig 2–1). This lateral lamella constitutes the lateral border of the olfactory fossa, with the lamina cribrosa providing its floor. The lateral lamina of the lamina cribrosa is also the medial wall of the dome of the ethmoid, its height and shape varying considerably from case to case. *It is critical to remember that the highest point of the roof of the ethmoid may be as much as 17 mm above the level of the lamina cribrosa.*

Because the structures of this portion of the roof of the ethmoid can vary so much in height, width, and shape, as well as from side to side, it is important that the surgeon has a thorough knowledge of the anatomy of this area before performing surgery. Only a good conventional or computed tomography (CT) radiogram, taken in the coronal plane, can provide the surgeon with adequate information about a patient's individual conditions, variations, and potential hazards (Fig 2–9).

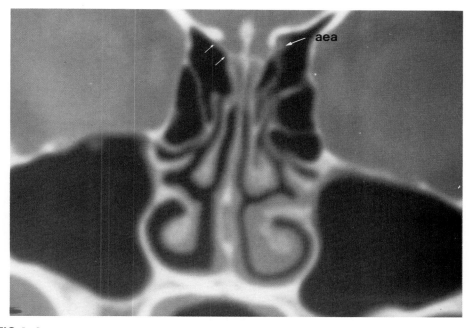

FIG 2–9.
This CT scan demonstrates the anatomy of the roof of the ethmoid. The thicker parts of the roof of the ethmoid, belonging to the frontal bone, can be distinguished from the thinner, medial wall of the ethmoid roof. The latter is formed by the lamina lateralis of the lamina cribrosa *(thin arrows on the right side).* Note on the left side the anterior ethmoidal artery *(arrow)* passing through the lateral lamella of the cribriform plate. *aea* = anterior ethmoidal artery.

The topographic relationships of the anterior ethmoidal artery are also especially important, because in its course from the orbit to the olfactory fossa, this vessel traverses three body cavities: the orbit, the ethmoidal labyrinth, and the anterior cranial fossa. Particularly at the point where the artery enters the anterior cranial fossa through the lateral lamella of the lamina cribrosa the surgeon encounters the most critical area of the entire anterior ethmoid sinus, and indeed of the entire anterior base of the skull. At this point the lateral lamella of the lamina cribrosa presents the least resistance to a probing instrument, being only 10% as strong as the roof of the ethmoid.

After its origin from the ophthalmic artery in the orbit, the anterior ethmoidal artery passes through the anterior ethmoidal foramen into the anterior ethmoid (Fig 2–10). It crosses the anterior ethmoid, surrounded only by a thin-walled bony channel (Fig 2–11). In some cases this ethmoidal canal is embedded in the roof of the ethmoid, particularly when the roof is very low and rises only slightly above the level of the lamina cribrosa. In most cases, however, the ethmoidal canal is connected to the roof of the ethmoid by a bony mesentery, with an interspace of as much as 5 mm. The point of insertion of this ethmoidal canal, also known as the orbitocranial canal, is usually directly behind the point where the roof of the ethmoid bends anterosuperiorly to form the posterosuperior border of the frontal recess. The first of the anterior ethmoidal cells reaching the lamina papyracea usually lies posterior to the ethmoidal canal. When the frontal sinus is absent, the anterior ethmoidal artery is usually located between the first and second of the ethmoidal cells that extend laterally to the lamina papyracea. In some texts these cells are referred to as the

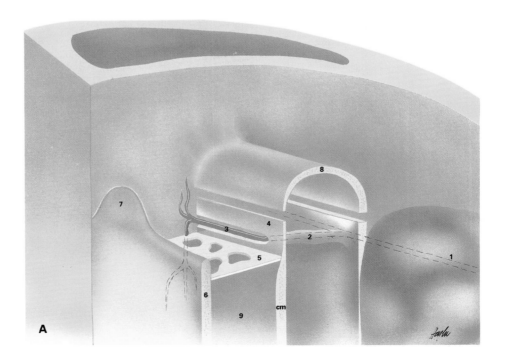

A

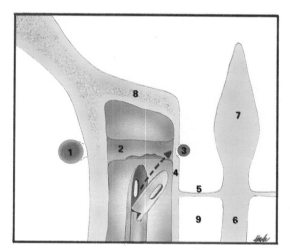

FIG 2–10.
Schematic drawing of the course of the anterior ethmoidal artery. For details, see text. The view is from medially behind and above toward the right anterior skull base. For **A** and **B,** *1* = ophthalmic artery in the orbit; *2* = anterior ethmoidal artery in the bony canal traversing the ethmoid; *3* = anterior ethmoidal artery after penetration of the lateral lamella of the cribriform plate in the "ethmoidal sulcus"; *4* = lateral lamella of the cribriform plate; *5* = cribriform plate; *6* = septum nasi; *7* = crista galli; *8* = frontal bone (providing the roof for the ethmoid; *9* = olfactory ridge of the common nasal meatus. **B,** an instrument is shown approaching the place of least resistance in the anterior skull base: the vicinity of the anterior ethmoidal artery in the ethmoidal sulcus.

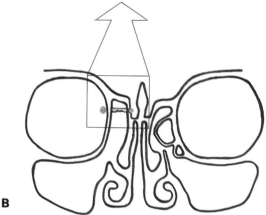

B

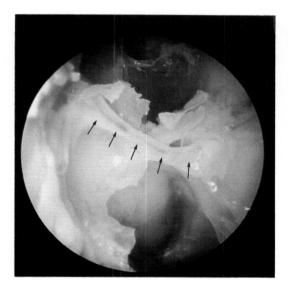

FIG 2–11.
Left anterior ethmoid artery on its way from the orbit to the olfactory fossa through the ethmoid as seen with a 30-degree lens. The course of the artery in its bony canal *(arrows)* can be seen clearly passing from right (the orbit) to left (the lateral lamella of the lamina cribrosa). The artery can be seen through the intact wall of its bony canal. The roof of the ethmoid can be seen behind the artery.

orbitoethmoidal cells. These points of reference can be seen only in an anatomic preparation in the sagittal plane from the medial side. They are of little assistance in an endoscopic surgical procedure that of necessity approaches the roof of the ethmoid from the front and below.

To identify the ethmoidal artery by the endoscopic approach, it is best to follow the anterior surface of the ethmoidal bulla in the direction of the roof of the ethmoid. If the bulla lamella extends up to the roof of the ethmoid, the ethmoidal artery can usually be found immediately adjacent to this point, usually 1 to 2 mm posteriorly. If the anterior bulla lamella does not extend to the roof of the ethmoid and there is no complete bony separation between frontal recess and the lateral sinus, the ethmoidal artery can be seen in the lateral sinus, depending somewhat on the configuration of the lateral sinus. The artery can sometimes be seen in the lateral sinus during diagnostic endoscopy, through a wide superior hiatus semilunaris, or more rarely from the frontal recess, without having to remove parts of the bulla.

After its occasionally sharply diagonal passage through the anterior ethmoid, the anterior ethmoidal artery reaches the olfactory fossa in the anterior cranial fossa by breaking through the lateral lamella of the lamina cribrosa (the lateral wall of the olfactory fossa). At this point the artery turns anteriorly in a groove of the lateral lamella, the so-called ethmoidal sulcus, where it gives off the anterior meningeal artery and finally reaches the nasal cavity through the cribroethmoidal foramen and the lamina cribrosa. In the nasal cavity it divides into the anterior nasal artery (with superior, lateral, and medial nasal branches), a posterior branch, and several small meningeal branches. This division into its terminal branches may take place before or after its passage through the lamina cribrosa.

The bony structures in the immediate vicinity of the anterior ethmoidal artery may show remarkable variation in thickness. Those parts of the roof of the ethmoid that are formed by the frontal bone are much thicker and stronger than the lateral wall of the olfactory fossa, which is formed by the lateral lamella of the lamina cribrosa (which equals the medial wall of the dome of the ethmoid). The frontal bone at the roof of the ethmoid has a mean thickness of 0.5 mm, whereas the lateral lamella averages only 0.2 mm. In the ethmoidal sulcus the thickness of the wall may be reduced to 0.05 mm. In this area, the bone is only 10% as strong as the rest of the roof of the ethmoid.

In a series of microdissections, Kainz established that the length of the ethmoidal sulcus is 3 to 10 mm on the left and 3 to 16 mm on the right. The length of the ethmoidal canal varies from 4 to 13 mm on the left and 5 to 15 mm on the right.

In 40% of cases the canal showed bony dehiscences that resulted in a partially or completely open canal. These dehiscences were usually located on the inferior side of the canal. There can be significant differences between the two sides in the same person. On one side the bony canal may be complete; on the other side the canal may be partially or completely open. In about 20% of the skulls that we studied, bony dehiscences were found on both sides.

The dura mater is only loosely attached to the skull. In the area of the olfactory fossa, however, the dura not only is thinner but also is firmly attached to the bone, particularly at the point where the anterior ethmoidal artery, its branches, and the olfactory filaments pass through the lamina cribrosa. In the majority of cases the anterior ethmoidal artery is intradural on its way through the olfactory fossa. In 29 of 40 skulls examined, the anterior ethmoidal artery was surrounded by dura from its entrance into the anterior ethmoidal canal all the way to the olfactory fossa. In eight skulls the artery entered the dura during its passage through the ethmoidal sulcus, and in three cases the artery was extradural along its entire course. In 75% the anterior ethmoidal artery consisted of a single vessel on both sides; in 15% there were two branches.

CLINICAL AND SURGICAL SIGNIFICANCE OF ANTERIOR ETHMOIDAL ARTERY AND DOME OF ETHMOID

In all forms of endonasal surgery, and particularly after blunt cranial trauma, the anterior ethmoidal artery and its immediate surroundings represent the point of least resistance. Fractures, hemorrhages, dural lesions, and all of their complications may occur in this area.

In blunt external trauma, fractures are most likely where there is a transition from thick bony segments to thinner ones. The lamina cribrosa and its lateral lamella are thus particularly prone to chip fractures. Because the dura is thin and firmly attached to the bone in this area, the anterior ethmoidal artery can be torn where it enters or leaves the olfactory fossa. Sharp bone fragments from the fracture site may puncture the dura and produce a persistent CSF fistula. The firm attachment of the dura may also lead to more extensive tears after blunt trauma, also producing a CSF fistula.

Tiny lesions caused by bone splinters that are undetectable even by high-resolution CT may permit entry of pathogens. In many cases, only repeated bouts of meningitis will suggest the presence of such microlesions resulting from prior trauma that may have occurred years previously and to which the patient attached no importance. When a fluorescein technique is used, these fistulas can usually be easily identified and located by endoscopy.

Because there may be dehiscences in the cranioorbital canal and also in the lamina cribrosa, the nasal mucosa may even normally lie in direct contact with the dura.

The olfactory filaments do not pass freely through the subarachnoid space, because they are surrounded from the olfactory bulb by a perineurium, which corresponds to the leptomeninges. Subsequently they pass through the subdural space and the dura.

Injuries to the base of the skull with dural lesions and ensuing CSF fistulas in the area of the roof of the anterior ethmoid are most likely to occur when the lateral lamella of the lamina cribrosa is particularly thin and high. This also applies to direct (iatrogenic) trauma. The danger area is not the highest point of the roof of the ethmoid, which is formed by the frontal bone and is ten times as strong as the lateral lamella of the lamina cribrosa in the area of the ethmoidal sulcus. The weakest point of the entire anterior base of the skull is that point at which the anterior ethmoidal artery leaves the ethmoid and proceeds anteriorly in the ethmoidal sulcus of the olfactory fossa. The surgeon must exercise the greatest caution when working under the roof of the ethmoid, in the vicinity of the anterior ethmoidal artery, and especially when turning the instruments medially. It is here that the thin bone of the lateral lamella provides the least resistance to the instrument and that the danger of a perforation into the olfactory fossa and thus into the anterior cranial fossa is greatest (see Fig 2–10, B).

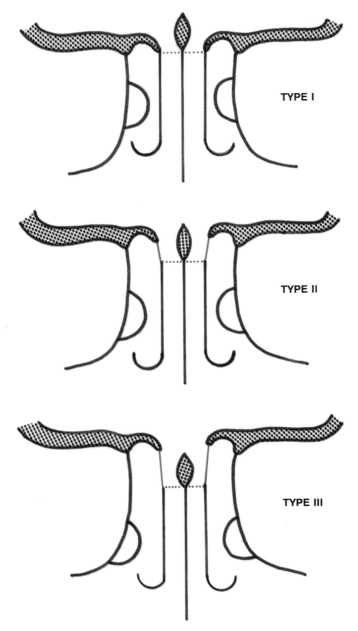

TYPE I

TYPE II

TYPE III

FIG 2–12.
Schematic drawing showing the three different types of olfactory fossa according to Keros. Note the length increases of the lateral lamellae of the cribriform plate from types I to III.

The configurations of the olfactory fossa have been classified by Keros into three types (Fig 2–12). In type I the olfactory fossa is flat, the roof of the ethmoid almost vertical, and the lateral lamella of the lamina cribrosa very short vertically. In type II the lateral lamella is longer, the course of the roof of the ethmoid steeper, and the olfactory fossa deeper. In type III the roof of the ethmoid is considerably higher than the lamina cribrosa, the lateral lamella particularly long and thin, and the olfactory fossa correspondingly deep. Type III is the most dangerous for the surgeon because of the likelihood of a perforation through the lateral lamella of the lamina cribrosa.

Perforations through the lamina cribrosa proper can best be avoided by staying strictly lateral to the insertion of the middle turbinate. When manipulations at the roof of the ethmoid become necessary, every attempt should be made to identify the anterior ethmoidal artery.

CLEFTS AND SPACES OF LATERAL NASAL WALL

The mucosal lining of the paranasal sinuses and of the primary nasal cavity not only is functional but also contributes to the shape of these areas. It is only after they are covered by the mucous membrane that the spaces and clefts of the ethmoid assume their definitive form and relationship to each other. Similarly, only after the maxillary sinus and the nasal passages are covered by mucous membrane do the nasal fontanelles become membranous components of the lateral nasal wall, and the natural ostium of the maxillary sinus assumes its definitive form only after it is lined by mucosa.

The clefts and spaces of the lateral nasal wall, which depend to a considerable degree on mucous membranes as far as their borders, extent, and pathophysiology are concerned, are discussed in this section.

Hiatus Semilunaris (Inferior Hiatus Semilunaris of Grünwald)

The term hiatus semilunaris was coined in 1880 by Zuckerkandl, who gave this name to both the cleft and the depression that was seen from a medial view between the free posterior margin of the uncinate process and the anterior surface of the ethmoidal bulla. The sickle-shaped hiatus semilunaris resembles a new moon. To avoid the long-standing confusion in terminology between the hiatus semilunaris and the various interpretations of the different infundibula (e.g., ethmoidal, maxillary, frontal), in this text we use the term hiatus semilunaris to refer to a strictly *two-dimensional formation*, namely, the sagittal cleft between the concave, free posterior border of the uncinate process and the convex, anterior surface of the ethmoidal bulla.

From the middle meatus, one can approach through this cleft a channel or pocket directed anteroinferiorly and superolaterally, designated as the ethmoidal infundibulum (see later discussion). The hiatus semilunaris (inferior) is thus the door through which we can reach the ethmoidal infundibulum.

Grünwald described a second hiatus semilunaris, the superior hiatus semilunaris, by which he meant the cleft that appears between the ethmoidal bulla and the middle meatus when there is a marked lateral sinus posterior to and above the ethmoidal bulla. The hiatus semilunaris superior is also a sickle-shaped cleft posteromedial to the ethmoidal bulla through which the lateral sinus can be probed. This cleft must not be confused with the turbinate sinus, which is a cleft in the sagittal plane, between a large ethmoidal bulla and a laterally curved middle turbinate that surrounds the bulla. Analogous to the relationship between the hiatus semilunaris inferior and the ethmoidal bulla, one can say that the turbinate sinus proceeds superiorly and laterally through the hiatus semilunaris superior to the lateral sinus when the latter is correspondingly pneumatized (Fig 2–13).

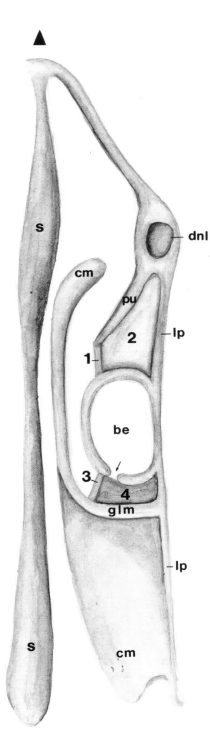

FIG 2–13.
On this horizontal (axial) section through a right lateral nasal wall, the relationships of some of the compartments of the anterior ethmoid are shown in a simplified schematic form. The proportions of the individual parts are intentionally distorted and exaggerated. The purpose of this drawing is to illustrate the principles of the topographic relationships. The view is toward a lateral nasal wall from above. The section is almost parallel to the hard palate, just above the horizontal portion of the ground lamella of the middle turbinate. The ground lamella is thus shown in its ascending, middle portion. The ethmoidal bulla is attached laterally to the lamina papyracea. The uncinate process inserts into the lateral nasal wall, directly behind the nasolacrimal duct. One reaches the ethmoidal infundibulum through the inferior hiatus semilunaris. The sinus lateralis is reached through the superior hiatus semilunaris. Note that the ethmoidal bulla normally opens into the lateral sinus *(arrow)*.

The position of the superior hiatus semilunaris is chosen somewhat arbitrarily. It cannot be nearly as accurately shown anatomically as can the position of the inferior hiatus semilunaris. Depending on the shape and depth of the lateral sinus and on the distance between the middle turbinate and the ethmoidal bulla, the cleft of the superior hiatus semilunaris can be placed slightly more medially or laterally. To indicate this range of position, we have not shown the superior hiatus semilunaris precisely in the sagittal plane.

The *black triangle* indicates the tip of the nose: *s* = nasal septum; *cm* = concha media; *glm* = ground lamella; *pu* = uncinate process; *dnl* = nasolacrimal duct; *lp* = lamina papyracea; *be* = bulla ethmoidalis; *1* = inferior hiatus semilunaris; *2* = ethmoidal infundibulum; *3* = superior hiatus semilunaris; *4* = sinus lateralis.

Ethmoidal Infundibulum

To avoid any misunderstanding, we use the term infundibulum to refer to one specific space in the anterior ethmoid, as described later. To clarify the topographic relationships, the term infundibulum should always be accompanied by the adjective "ethmoidal."

The ethmoidal infundibulum is a cleftlike *three-dimensional space* in the lateral wall of the nose that belongs to the anterior ethmoid. The medial wall of this space is provided by in the entire extent of the uncinate process and its mucosal covering. The major part of the lateral wall of the ethmoidal infundibulum is provided by the lamina papyracea of the orbit, with the frontal process of the maxilla and in rare cases the lacrimal bone providing the remainder of its lateral wall anterosuperiorly. The anterior border of the uncinate process fuses with the bones of the lateral nasal wall at a sharp angle and provides a bony connection inferiorly with the inferior turbinate. Bony defects in this area are covered by dense connective tissue (periosteum) and mucous membrane and are thus closed in the area of the anterior (inferior) nasal fontanelle. Through the line of attachment of the anterior margin of the uncinate process to the lateral nasal wall, the ethmoidal infundibulum ends blindly anteriorly in an acute angle. This is the reason that the lumen of the ethmoidal infundibulum appears to be V shaped in a horizontal section (e.g., axial CT; see Fig 2–13).

If the middle turbinate is reflected superiorly in an anatomic preparation (Fig 2–14), the previously described structures can be seen. The posterior, free margin of the uncinate process, which bends slightly medially, is evident. The anterior insertion of the uncinate process cannot be identified, because it is covered by a layer of mucosa continuous with that of the lateral nasal wall. Occasionally a slight depression (sulcus) can be seen along the line where the uncinate process arises from the lateral nasal wall.

Between the anterior margin of the ethmoidal bulla and the free posterior margin of the uncinate process is the two-dimensional hiatus semilunaris (see Fig 2–14, A–C). Through the hiatus semilunaris, anteriorly, inferiorly, and

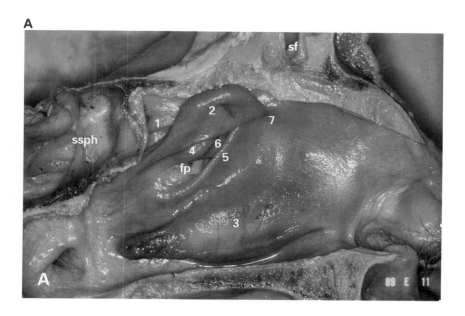

B

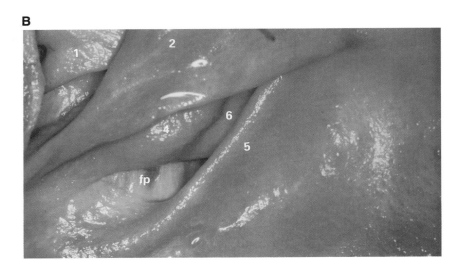

C

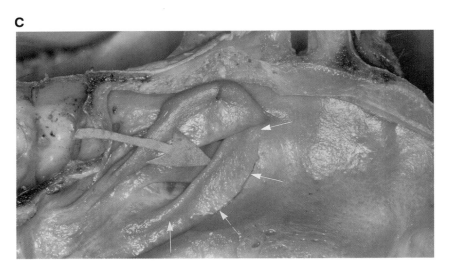

D

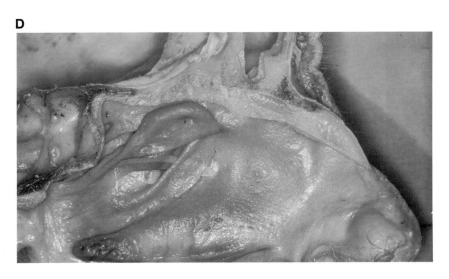

E

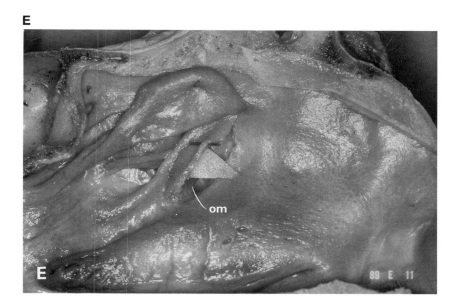

F

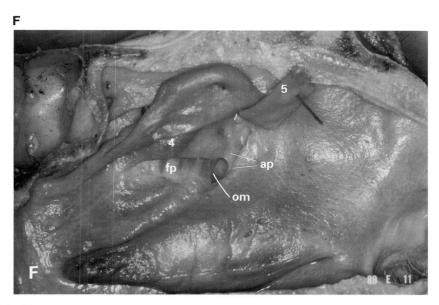

FIG 2–14.
Cadaveric anatomic preparation displaying the ethmoidal infundibulum in the lateral nasal wall. The middle turbinate has been reflected superiorly for demonstration purposes. **A,** overview. Key to **A** to **F:** *1* = superior turbinate; *2* = middle turbinate; *3* = inferior turbinate; *4* = ethmoidal bulla; *5* = uncinate process; *6* = hiatus semilunaris; *7* = agger nasi; *sf* = frontal sinus; *ssph* = sphenoid sinus; *fp* = posterior nasal fontanelle; *om* = maxillary sinus ostium; *fa* = anterior nasal fontanelle. **B,** close-up view. **C,** incision through the anterior attachment of the uncinate process is indicated by the *small arrows. Red arrow* shows the way into the ethmoidal infundibulum. **D,** *red arrow* is shown appearing through the anterior attachment of the uncinate process (out of the anterior blind end of the ethmoidal infundibulum. **E,** hidden position of the maxillary sinus ostium at the floor of the middle to posterior third of the ethmoidal infundibulum. **F,** uncinate process has been resected inferiorly and folded upward, displaying the lateral wall of the ethmoidal infundibulum.

superiorly, a cleftlike hollow space, the ethmoidal infundibulum (see Fig 2–14, A–C), which ends anteriorly in a sharp angle (corresponding to the line of attachment of the uncinate process to the lateral nasal wall), can be entered. Medially this space is bordered along its entire length by the uncinate process with its mucosal lining. The lateral wall of the ethmoidal infundibulum is composed primarily of the lamina papyracea of the orbit, with some participation by the frontal process of the maxilla and rarely by the lacrimal bone. Further inferiorly and posteriorly the lateral wall of the ethmoidal infundibulum is formed by the mucosa-covered connective tissue components of the posterior nasal fontanelle.

The posterior border of the ethmoidal infundibulum is composed largely of the anterior surface of the ethmoidal bulla, in front of which the infundibulum opens into the middle meatus through the hiatus semilunaris. Depending on the structure of the uncinate process, in its most superior portion the relationship of the ethmoidal infundibulum to the base of the skull and to the frontal recess may vary (Fig 2–15; see later discussion).

A schematic cast of the ethmoidal infundibulum would have the shape of an orange slice, with the difference that the wide side is posterior (i.e., on the concave side) and the thinner convex side terminates in a pointed corner. The hiatus semilunaris can be taken for the door through which the ethmoidal infundibulum can be entered from the posteromedial side.

It must be noted that in most cases it is not possible to view the maxillary sinus ostium by looking into the middle meatus. The ostia seen with the endoscope in the middle meatus are almost always accessory, located either in the anterior or posterior fontanelle. Figure 2–14, E and F shows clearly how the natural ostium of the maxillary sinus is hidden deeply in the ethmoidal infundibulum.

Figure 2–14, D and E demonstrates how a probe can be passed through the hiatus semilunaris behind the uncinate process and become visible again at the line of insertion of the uncinate process into the lateral nasal wall. The insertion of the uncinate process has been transected during the dissection. The hidden part of the probe lies within the ethmoidal infundibulum. Only when the uncinate process is displaced medially and posteriorly (Fig 2–14, F) can the position and size of the natural ostium of the maxillary sinus be seen. The natural ostium can usually be found at the transition from the middle to the posterior segment of the ethmoidal infundibulum at its floor. These relationships can be more clearly seen when the uncinate process is severed from its inferior insertion and folded superiorly (Fig 2–14, F).

This preparation demonstrates the extent to which the ostium of the maxillary sinus, and therefore the maxillary sinus itself, depends on the condition of the ethmoidal infundibulum, the hiatus semilunaris, and adjacent middle meatus. Inflammatory processes in any of these areas can easily spread to the adjacent areas and involve the hiatus semilunaris and the ethmoidal infundibulum. If the hiatus semilunaris or the ethmoidal infundibulum areas are partially or completely obstructed, the maxillary sinus will become poorly ventilated and secretions will be retained in the maxillary sinus.

Superiorly the configuration of the ethmoidal infundibulum, and therefore its relationship to the frontal recess, depends largely on the behavior of the uncinate process. As shown in Figure 2–15, if the uncinate process bends laterally in its uppermost portion and inserts into the lamina papyracea, the ethmoidal infundibulum is closed superiorly by a blind pouch called the recessus terminalis (terminal recess). In this case, the ethmoidal infundibulum

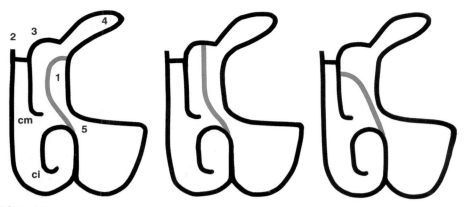

FIG 2–15.
Schematic drawings of uncinate process variations (in *red*) show their impact on the relationship of the frontal recess and the ethmoidal infundibulum. *1* = ethmoidal infundibulum; *2* = frontal recess; *3* = frontal sinus ostium; *4* = frontal sinus; *5* = maxillary sinus ostium; *cm* = concha media; *ci* = concha inferior.

and the frontal recess are separated from each other so that the frontal recess opens into the middle meatus medial to the ethmoidal infundibulum between the uncinate process and the middle turbinate; the route of drainage and ventilation of the frontal sinus runs medial to the ethmoidal infundibulum.

The uncinate process can also extend directly superiorly and either extend to the roof of the ethmoid or gradually taper anteriorly. It can also turn medially and fuse with the middle turbinate. In the last two situations (see Fig 2–15), the frontal recess and consequently the frontal sinus open directly into the ethmoidal infundibulum. This is important in the spread of inflammatory processes.

If the ethmoidal infundibulum has a terminal recess, the separation from the frontal recess makes involvement of the latter less likely. Similarly, a disease in the frontal recess is not so likely to spread to the ethmoidal infundibulum and thus involve the maxillary sinus secondarily.

So far, the structure of the ethmoidal infundibulum has been presented in schematic form; in life, numerous variations occur.

The superior, bony end of the uncinate process may become divided into three branches that insert into the base of the skull, the lamina papyracea, and the middle turbinate. Depending on the development of these branches, various septations or inlets may be formed. The mucosal lining membrane may produce partial or complete septation of the terminal recess and the formation of an additional blind pouch at the base of the skull or at the middle turbinate. In Figure 2–14 a number of clearly visible slight indentations can be seen in the lateral wall of the ethmoidal infundibulum when the uncinate process is deflected upward. These can expand anteriorly in varying numbers and sizes and evolve into the so-called infundibular cells. If such a cell develops anteriorly and superiorly, it can extend as far as the lacrimal bone and may be called an ethmolacrimal cell. The agger nasi may become pneumatized from the frontal recess (see later discussion). Agger nasi cells also have the lacrimal bone as their lateral wall. If both ethmolacrimal and agger nasi cells are present simultaneously, it may be difficult, if not impossible, to sort them out accurately through the endoscope. This is particularly true when the cells are diseased.

Finally, the uncinate process may itself become pneumatized and cause significant narrowing of the ethmoidal infundibulum and middle meatus.

Posteriorly the ethmoidal infundibulum tapers parallel to the tapering of the uncinate process. Depending on the form of the uncinate process, the entire length of the ethmoidal infundibulum may reach 4 cm. Its greatest depth (measured vertically against the free, posterior margin of the uncinate process) may be as much as 12 mm, and its greatest width (free margin of the uncinate process to the lamina papyracea) 5 to 6 mm. The latter occurs primarily when the uncinate process is bent medially or is doubled back anteriorly.

It is important for the surgeon to remember that the ethmoidal infundibulum may in some patients be very shallow (i.e., the uncinate process) during its entire length and is never farther from the lamina papyracea than 1 to 1.5 mm. The ethmoidal infundibulum may be almost atelectatic, when anatomic variations (e.g., paradoxically bent middle meatus, concha bullosa, or in the presence of a hypoplastic maxillary sinus) or pathologic processes compress the uncinate process laterally against the lamina papyracea.

Frontal Recess

The name and description of the space that, following Killian, we call the frontal recess of the anterior ethmoid has in the past been confusing. It has been called the nasal part of the frontal sinus, the frontal infundibulum, and the nasofrontal duct, and has even been equated with the ethmoidal infundibulum.

We follow Killian's terminology for good reason, because from a developmental point of view this space is the superior continuation of the ascending branch of the first primary, interturbinal furrow, namely, the groove between the first and second ethmoidal turbinates. The descending branch of this first furrow becomes the ethmoidal infundibulum, indicating the close topographic relationship between these two structures (see Fig 2–14). The frontal sinus originates from the anterosuperior pneumatization of the frontal recess into the frontal bone.

The term nasofrontal duct suggests a tubular bony structure that in reality exists only in the rarest of cases, as a connecting link between the anterior ethmoid and the frontal sinus. The ostium of the frontal sinus is formed only when the frontal bone becomes attached to the ethmoid and when the immediate margins of the ostium of the frontal sinus are provided by parts of the ethmoid. If we examine a sagittal section of an anatomic preparation and look at the transition from the frontal sinus to the ethmoid (Fig 2–16), we can see that the medial part of the floor of the frontal sinus is shaped like a funnel, with its narrow end directed toward the ostium. Inferior to the ostium, in the area of the ethmoid, is another funnel-shaped space, the frontal recess, that widens from its narrowest point at the frontal ostium in a sagittal downward direction. In a sagittal section, therefore, there is an hourglass-shaped structure, with its narrowest part (the waist) located at the frontal ostium and the lower part designated as the frontal recess. Its limits, shape, and width are determined largely by its neighboring structures (see Fig 2–16).

The medial border of the frontal recess is almost always the lateral surface of the most anterior portion of the middle turbinate. Only when the uncinate process is markedly bent medially and also fused with the insertion of the middle turbinate does the most anterosuperior part of the uncinate process serve in a small area as the medial wall of the frontal recess (see Fig 2–15). The lamina papyracea forms a large part of the lateral wall of the frontal recess with its most anterosuperior extension. If the ethmoidal infundibulum has a terminal recess (Fig 2–15), the uncinate process forms part of the *lateral* wall and also contributes to the floor of the frontal recess in its most anterior aspects. The roof of the frontal recess is made up of those parts of the frontal bone that form the roof of the ethmoid with their ethmoidal foveolae. On the way anteriorly they bend slightly superiorly from their horizontal orientation and ultimately become the posterior wall of the frontal sinus.

The frontal ostium is usually found in the most anterosuperior part of the frontal recess.

The posterior wall of the frontal recess can be a single unit if the ground lamella of the ethmoidal bulla ascends in continuity and along its entire width to the roof of the ethmoid. In this case the ground lamella of the ethmoidal bulla separates the frontal recess from the lateral sinus (if there is one). Because the bulla lamella is frequently only incomplete and reaches the roof of the ethmoid only with some branches or not at all, the frontal recess may communicate widely posteriorly with a space above (and occasionally behind) the ethmoidal bulla, namely, the lateral sinus. Some rudimental frontal ridges may exist in the

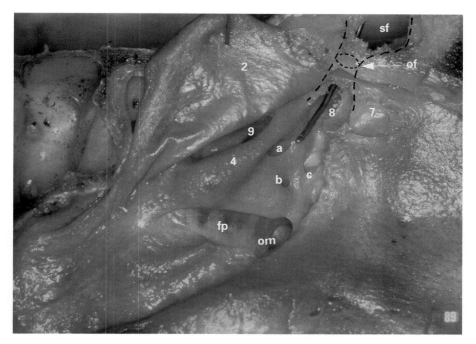

FIG 2–16.
Anatomic preparation showing the frontal recess after total resection of the uncinate. A probe has been passed from the frontal sinus into the frontal recess. *Dotted line* demonstrates the hourglass shape of the frontal recess toward the sinus ostium and floor. A small agger nasi cell is present, pneumatized from the frontal recess. In this case, the frontal recess passes directly into the ethmoidal infundibulum (see Fig 2–15, types II and III). Also clearly visible in this case is the lateral sinus between the bulla and ground lamella of the middle turbinate. The semilunar cleft through which the lateral sinus can be entered from medially and inferiorly is the hiatus semilunaris superior. *2* = middle turbinate; *4* = ethmoidal bulla; *7* = agger nasi; *8* = frontal recess; *9* = lateral sinus; *a, b,* and *c* = indentations and small recesses in the lateral wall of the infundibulum; *sf* = frontal sinus; *of* = area of the frontal sinus ostium; *fp* = posterior nasal fontanelle; *om* = maxillary sinus ostium.

frontal recess as smaller or larger, mostly transverse bony ridges. They extend from the roof of the ethmoid in the frontal plane downward, and may also serve as the posterior wall of the frontal recess.

Depending on the position of the uncinate process, the frontal recess may open into the middle meatus, medial to the uncinate process between the uncinate process and the middle turbinate or directly into the ethmoidal infundibulum (see Fig 2–15).

The shape of the bulla lamella can affect the configuration of the frontal recess to a large extent. If it extends far forward and the bulla is well developed, the frontal recess will be narrowed. If there is also marked pneumatization of the agger nasi and additional frontal ethmoidal cells, the frontal recess may be narrowed to a small passage or even to a tubular lumen. It is this configuration that probably gave rise to the term nasofrontal duct. But even when there is such a tubular configuration, it must be remembered that this is not an independent bony structure but simply a recess located between other independent bony structures.

The anatomic situation can be further complicated in that the most anterior ethmoidal cells may develop from the frontal recess. Thus pneumatization of the agger nasi may begin here. The middle turbinate can also become pneumatized from the frontal recess. Cells not uncommonly develop in the frontal bone, alongside the frontal sinus. Zuckerkandl called these the bulla frontalis. This variation may range from a bare suggestion of a bulge of the frontal recess into the floor of the frontal sinus to the formation of two or more approximately equally large cells on one side of the frontal bone. All of these cells open into the frontal recess. In some cases it may become impossible to determine which of the cells is the true frontal sinus and which is the bulla frontalis.

It therefore makes no sense from the perspective of the endoscopic diagnostician or surgeon to attempt to give a name or an anatomic or topographic designation to every single recess or inlet that can be seen with a 30- or 70-degree lens under the insertion of the middle turbinate (Fig 2–17), yet this attempt is made all the time.

The relationships of the uncinate process are too uncertain, particularly when there are pathologic mucous membrane changes or polyps present, and

A

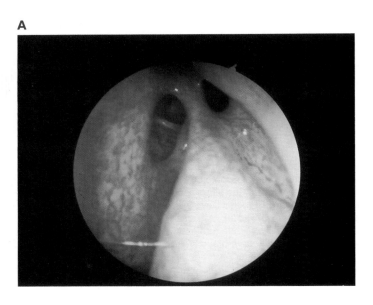

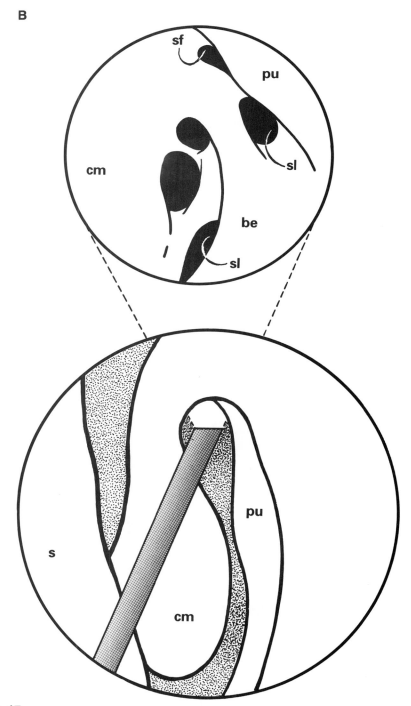

FIG 2–17.
A, endoscopic view into a frontal recess on a left side. (30-degree lens.) **B,** schematic diagram of the approach to the frontal recess and the view through the endoscope seen in **A.** *sf* = frontal sinus; *sl* = lateral sinus; *pu* = uncinate process; *be* = ethmoidal bulla; *cm* = concha media; *s* = septum.

can be really identified only after careful surgical dissection (Fig 2–18). Only rarely and when the access is very broad can a direct view into the frontal sinus be obtained and this sinus differentiated from extensive frontal cell formation with supraorbital extension. Without a good CT scan the various access routes to the frontal sinus can be identified endoscopically only in the ideal case and when there is no pathologic condition in the ethmoid. In cases of disease, probability and clinical experience may allow certain more or less accurate conclusions, but absolute certainty can be obtained only after careful surgical dissection.

Lateral Sinus

The space designated by Grünwald as the sinus lateralis is not a constant feature. When extensively pneumatized, it may extend above and beyond the ethmoidal bulla. Its borders include the lamina papyracea laterally, the roof of the ethmoid superiorly, the ground lamella of the middle turbinate posteriorly, and the roof and posterior wall of the ethmoidal bulla anteriorly and inferiorly (see Fig 2–18). When a lateral sinus is well pneumatized, the ethmoidal bulla usually opens into it.

If the ground lamella of the ethmoidal bulla extends only partially or not at all to the roof of the ethmoid, the lateral sinus may continue anteriorly into the frontal recess. The lateral sinus can be reached through the superior hiatus semilunaris medially between the ethmoidal bulla and the middle turbinate.

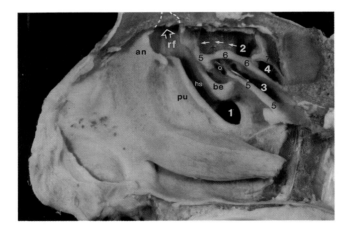

FIG 2–18.
Dissection of a right lateral nasal wall showing the frontal recess opening directly into the ethmoidal infundibulum, lateral to the uncinate process. *Outlined arrow* points to the ostium of the frontal sinus. *Dotted lines* indicate the cranial contour of the frontal recess as far as the ostium of the frontal sinus, which lies just at the edge of the illustration. A small cell has developed from the frontal recess into the agger nasi. The medial wall of the sinus lateralis (+) corresponds to the ground lamella of the middle turbinate, bulging far posteriorly. This posterior bulge was caused by a well-developed sinus lateralis. During the dissection, it was opened from the medial side (o), and a sound was placed into the superior meatus from the sinus lateralis through a dehiscence in the ground lamella. *1* = large accessory ostium in the posterior fontanelle; *2* = posterior ethmoidal cell, extending anteriorly, medial to the sinus lateralis (*white arrows*); *3* = superior meatus; *4* = supreme meatus; *5* = line of resection of the middle turbinate; *6* = superior turbinate (lower margin of the resection: a view into the posterior ethmoid is possible through the window, 2); *7* = supreme turbinate; *an* = agger nasi; *rf* = frontal recess; *hs* = hiatus semilunaris (inferior); *be* = ethmoidal bulla; *pu* = uncinate process.

3 Imaging of Paranasal Sinuses

Katherine Evans, M.D.
Lalitha Shankar, M.D.

The Messerklinger technique of functional endoscopic sinus surgery is first and foremost a diagnostic concept that relies on two primary and equally important diagnostic modalities: endoscopic examination of the nasal cavities and tomographic examination of the nasal cavity and paranasal sinuses. Noninvasive diagnostic endoscopy has its limits, and the deeper structures cannot be evaluated by endoscopy alone. Computed tomography (CT) and endoscopy thus compliment each other in the assessment of the individual patient.

The anterior ethmoidal sinuses and the ostiomeatal complex are the primary sites of the mucosal pathologic conditions responsible for chronic infection in the major paranasal sinuses. The ethmoidal infundibulum, the hiatus semilunaris, and the middle meatus are the channels through which the frontal, maxillary, and anterior ethmoidal air cells drain. Swelling or apposition of the adjacent mucociliary surfaces may result in poor ventilation and obstruction to drainage of the larger paranasal sinuses. Any anatomic variants present in this region, trauma, or hyperplasia of the mucosa from previous infections can narrow these critical channels, impairing drainage from and ventilation of the larger paranasal sinuses, thereby producing chronic sinusitis.

CT of the paranasal sinuses is indispensable in identifying disease that may not be appreciated during routine clinical examination either with the nasal speculum or even by detailed endoscopic examination. This is particularly true in disease involving solely the ostiomeatal complex or the posterior ethmoidal and sphenoidal sinuses. In these areas CT is extremely valuable because unsuspected advanced mucosal disease can be effectively demonstrated by high-resolution CT (HRCT). CT of the paranasal sinuses should be considered a mandatory investigation for assessing the presence or absence of pathologic conditions of the paranasal sinuses when recurrent medical treatment has failed. In addition, CT examination of the paranasal sinuses will provide an anatomic road map of the paranasal sinuses and identify the presence of significant anatomic abnormalities, the location and severity of the disease, and the exact location of the obstruction.

CONVENTIONAL RADIOGRAPHS

1. Caldwell projection
2. Lateral projection
3. Water's projection
4. Submentovertex projection

43

These radiographic films are adequate only for preliminary assessment of the paranasal sinuses. The anterior ethmoidal sinuses, upper nasal cavity, and frontal recess are poorly demonstrated in these views. In many patients with significant ostiomeatal complex disease, which can be identified on HRCT, detailed examination of their conventional radiographs may reveal no abnormalities.

In cases of acute sinusitis, plain radiographs are usually sufficient, and for follow-up a repeat Water's view is generally appropriate. In some centers, the use of ultrasound for the identification of fluid within the maxillary or frontal sinuses has gained popularity. The loss of the ultrasonic back wall echo is considered to indicate improvement in the state of the sinus.

CORONAL COMPUTED TOMOGRAPHY

Preliminary coronal CT or polytomography of the paranasal sinuses is mandatory prior to functional endoscopic sinus surgery to permit safe performance of the surgical procedure. The surgeon and the radiologist must understand clearly the normal and pathologic anatomy in this region.

Technique

Coronal scans (Table 3–1) are preferred because the anatomy and pathology are examined in a plane almost identical to that approached by the endoscopist. Figures 3–1 to 3–10 illustrate the frontal sinus anteriorly to the sphenoidal sinus posteriorly. If there is any doubt about its adequacy for a complete examination, scans in the axial plane (Table 3–2) are also done. Axial scans from the level of the hard palate to the cribriform fossa are shown in Figures 3–11 to 3–20.

Parameters for Coronal CT Scans

Patient position	Prone or supine
Gantry angulation	Perpendicular to infraorbitomeatal line
Section thickness	4-mm slices
Table increment	3 or 4 mm each step (3-mm step is necessary if three-dimensional CT reconstruction is to be performed)
Scan limits	From posterior margin of sphenoidal sinus to frontal sinus
kV peak:	125
mamp/sec	450

Parameters for Axial CT scans

Patient position	Supine
Gantry position	Parallel to orbitomeatal line
Scan limits	From alveolar ridge to top of frontal sinus

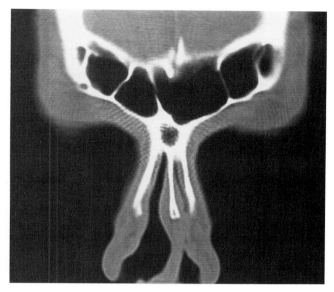

FIG 3–1.
Septation of a normal frontal sinus. Coronal scan of the frontal sinuses demonstrates a multiseptated frontal sinus, normal nasal bones, and anterior deviation of the cartilaginous nasal septum to the left.

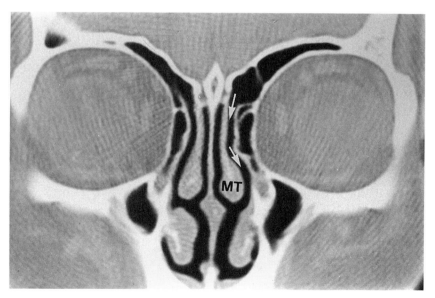

FIG 3–2.
Normal frontal recess. Scan demonstrates a normal, wide, patent frontal recess *(upper arrow)*. In this patient the frontal recess drains directly into the middle meatus *(lower arrow)*. Vertical insertion of the middle turbinate *(MT)* can be clearly seen.

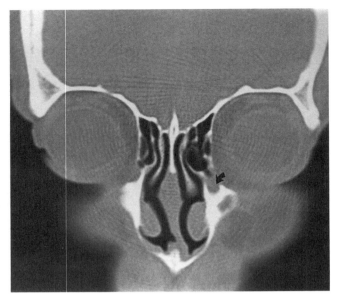

FIG 3–3.
Lacrimal fossa. Soft-density shadow of the lacrimal sac *(arrows)* is demonstrated at the inferomedial aspect of the orbit.

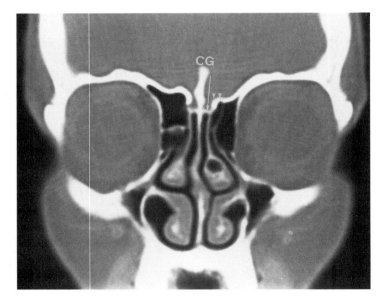

FIG 3–4.
Cribriform plate. Fovea ethmoidalis can clearly be seen to be both higher *(arrowhead)* and thicker than the cribriform plate *(arrow)*. This demonstrates the hazards of surgery in this area. Note the bony channel for the anterior ethmoidal artery on the right. Crista galli is also demonstrated *(CG)*. Other findings include bilateral bony hypertrophy of the middle turbinates and a small air cell in the left middle turbinate (concha bullosa).

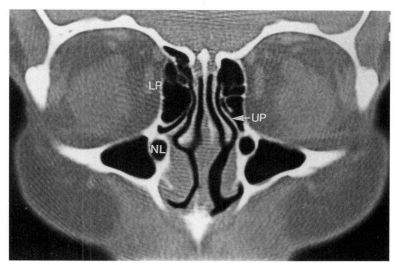

FIG 3–5.
Nasolacrimal duct. Anterior coronal scan demonstrates air in both nasolacrimal ducts *(NL)*. Nasolacrimal duct is bounded by the maxilla, the lacrimal bone, and the inferior turbinate. Both uncinate processes *(UP)* are elongated. Note the intimate relationship between the origin of the uncinate processes and the nasolacrimal duct. *LP* = thin lamina papyracea.

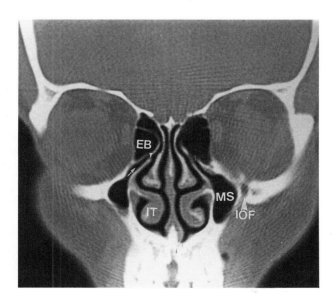

FIG 3–6.
Normal maxillary sinus. Scan demonstrates the anterior portion of the maxillary sinus *(MS)* draining through the maxillary ostia into the ethmoidal infundibulum *(arrow)*. Infundibulum channel is bounded superolaterally by the ethmoidal bulla *(EB)* and inferomedially by the uncinate process *(UP)*. Ethmoidal infundibulum opens into the hiatus semilunaris. Hiatus semilunaris is a two-dimensional slitlike opening that connects the infundibulum to the middle meatus *(arrowhead)*. *IOF* = infraorbital foramen, *IT* = inferior turbinate.

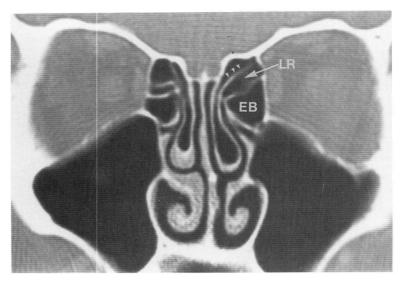

FIG 3–7.
Lateral recess. Coronal scan demonstrates bilateral concha bullosa. Horizontal insertion of the left middle turbinate *(arrowheads)* is seen. Space between the posterior margin of the ethmoidal bulla *(EB)* and the horizontal insertion of the middle turbinate is the lateral recess *(LR)*.

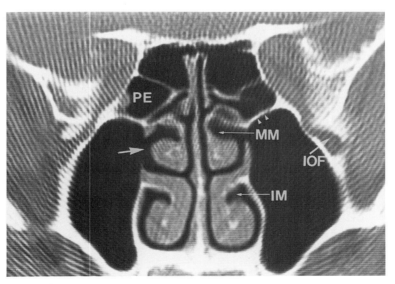

FIG 3–8.
Accessory maxillary ostia. Coronal scan of the posterior ethmoid air cells *(PE)* and the maxillary sinus demonstrates a large accessory maxillary sinus ostium on the right *(arrow)* just lateral to the middle turbinate, and a smaller one on the left close to the posterior part of the middle meatus *(NM)*. Thin plate of bone separating the superomedial margin of the maxillary sinus from the posterior ethmoidal air cells is the ethmomaxillary plate *(arrowheads)*. IOF = inferior orbital fissure, IM = inferior meatus.

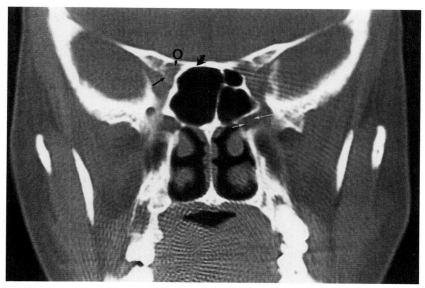

FIG 3–9.
Sphenoidal sinus. Sphenoethmoidal recess communicates with the pterygopalatine fossa through the sphenopalatine foramen *(between white arrows)*. Optic foramen *(O)* is separated from the superior orbital fissure by the optic strut *(black arrow)*. Planum sphenoidale of the lesser wing of the sphenoidal sinus is also demonstrated *(curved black arrow)*.

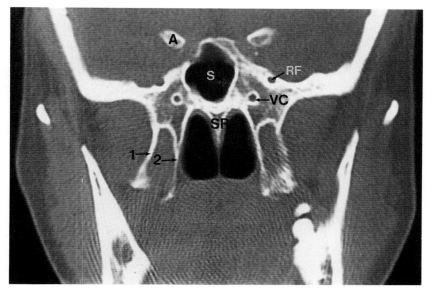

FIG 3–10.
Sphenoidal sinus. Scan demonstrates the sphenoid sinus *(S)*, foramen rotundum *(RF)*, vidian canal *(VC)*, anterior clinoid process *(A)*, sphenoid rostrum *(SR)*, and lateral *(1)* and medial *(2)* pterygoid plates bordering the pterygoid fossa.

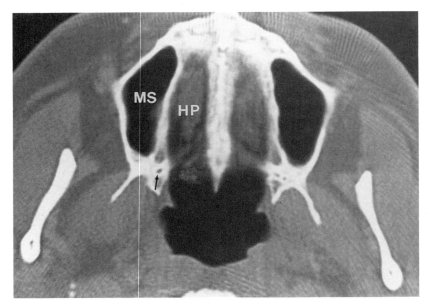

FIG 3–11.
Normal axial scan demonstrates a section through the hard palate *(HP)* and the alveolar recesses of the maxillary sinuses *(MS)*. Palatine foramina that transmit the greater and lesser palatine nerves are also shown *(arrow)*.

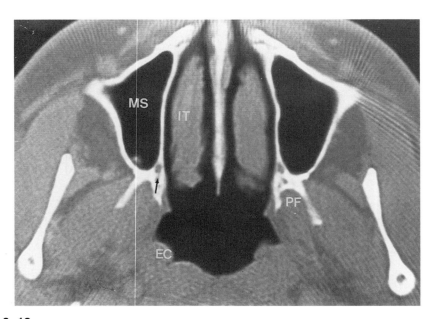

FIG 3–12.
Normal axial scan demonstrates the maxillary sinuses *(MS)* and the inferior turbinate *(IT)*. Posterior to the maxillary sinus lie the medial and lateral pterygoid plates, which enclose the pterygoid fossa *(PF)*. Palatine canals are shown *(arrow)*. Eustachian cushion *(EC)* is shown protruding into the nasopharynx.

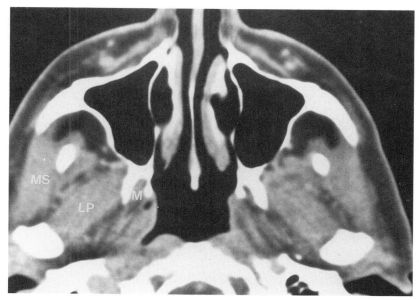

FIG 3–13.
Normal axial scan. This narrow window axial scan demonstrates the muscles of mastication: lateral pterygoid *(LP)*, medial pterygoid *(M)*, and masseter *(MS)*. These muscles are clearly separated by fat planes.

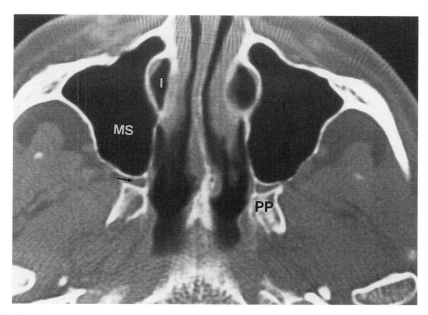

FIG 3–14.
Normal axial scan demonstrates the maxillary sinus *(MS)*, pterygopalatine fossa *(black arrow)*, and pterygoid process *(PP)*. Superior aspect of the inferior meatus *(I)* is transected in this view.

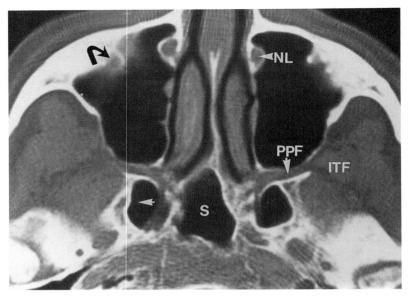

FIG 3–15.
Normal axial scan demonstrates the pterygopalatine fossa *(PPF)* communicating laterally with the infratemporal fossa *(ITF)* and medially with the nasal cavity through the sphenopalatine foramen. Nasolacrimal duct *(NL)*, inferior orbital nerve *(curved arrow)*, and an accessory maxillary sinus ostium are demonstrated. Pterygoid plates are pneumatized *(arrow)*, usually from the sphenoidal sinus *(S)*.

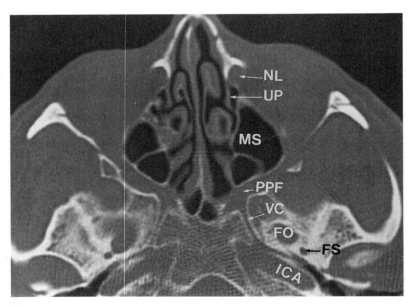

FIG 3–16.
Normal axial scan demonstrates the uncinate process *(UP)* arising close to the wall of the nasolacrimal duct *(NL)*. Also demonstrated are the vidian canal *(VC)*, foramen ovale *(FO)*, foramen spinosum *(FS)*, and pterygopalatine fossa *(PPF)*, continuing laterally as the infraorbital fissure. The maxillary sinus *(MS)* and internal carotid artery *(ICA)* are also shown.

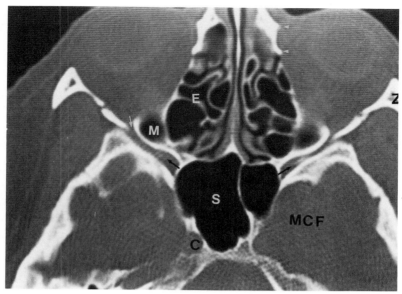

FIG 3–17.
Normal axial scan demonstrates the anterior and posterior lacrimal crests *(arrowheads)*, ethmoid labyrinth *(E)*, superior recess of the maxillary sinus *(M)*, zygoma *(Z)*, pterygopalatine fossa *(black arrow)*, inferior orbital foramen *(white arrow)*, middle cranial fossa *(MCF)*, sphenoidal sinus *(S)*, and internal carotid artery *(C)*.

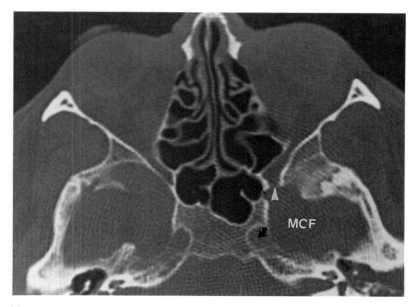

FIG 3–18.
Normal axial scan demonstrates the foramen rotundum *(white arrow)*, middle cranial fossa *(MCF)*, and internal carotid artery *(curved black arrow)*.

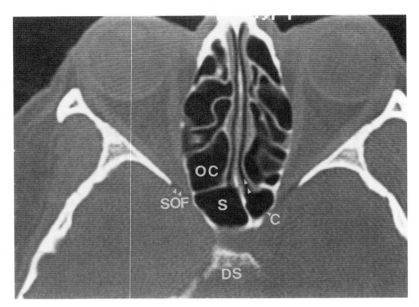

FIG 3–19.
Normal axial scan demonstrates the posterior ethmoid Onodi cell *(OC)*, superior orbital fissure *(SOF)*, sphenoidal sinus *(S)*, sphenoid sinus ostium *(arrowheads)*, impression of the internal carotid artery *(C)*, and dorsum sella *(DS)*.

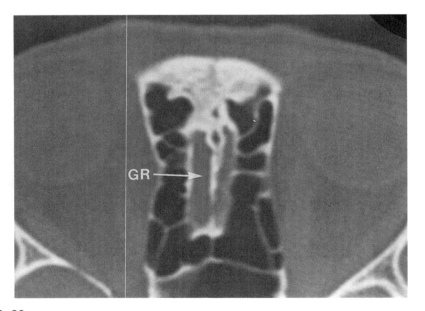

FIG 3–20.
Axial scan shows the location of the gyrus rectus *(GR)* of the frontal lobe. Note how the ethmoidal air cells rise above this portion of the frontal lobe.

The scanner raw data are transiently saved, and the bone and soft tissues are visualized with the appropriate window settings. For routine CT of the paranasal sinuses, the scanner is set with a wide window setting of 2000 centered around -250; this setting will usually demonstrate adequately both bone and soft tissue. When soft tissue pathologic conditions are to be emphasized, the scanner is set with a window of 300, centered at $+65$. The narrow window settings assist in characterizing tumors. If there is significant involvement of the surrounding soft tissue with loss of the fat plane, the lesion is more likely malignant. This situation can be more accurately assessed with narrow window settings. The bone window settings are excellent for assessment of bony erosion or destruction.

Indications for scanning in the axial plane include:

1. Tumors.
2. Trauma. (both axial and coronal plane scans are required in these situations.)
3. Children and elderly or uncooperative patients in whom positioning for coronal CT is difficult.

Secondary reconstruction in the coronal plane can be performed if necessary. Multiplanar scanning is ideal; however, time, patient compliance, increased radiation dose, and cost restrict the use of this more extensive examination in patients with benign disease.

INTRAVENOUS CONTRAST ADMINISTRATION

Intravenous contrast administration is at the discretion of the radiologist. The indications include:

1. Malignant tumors.
2. Vascular abnormalities. The vascularity of the lesion and its relationship to the major vessels can be assessed preoperatively. An angiogram also serves as a road map if embolization is being contemplated.
3. Inflammatory sinus disease in which complications such as abscess, thrombosis, or intracranial or intraorbital spread of infection are suspected.

The intravenous contrast medium used is a nonionic agent such as Omnipaque or Isovue (80 mL), optimally administered by an automatic injector at a rate of 1 mL/sec, followed by a 25- to 30-second delay.

Advantages

1. The administration of intravenous contrast medium helps to distinguish between active and chronic inflammatory disease. Mucosal enhancement is visible in active inflammation.
2. The distinction between allergic and inflammatory polyps on a CT scan can be helped by the administration of intravenous contrast medium. Inflammatory polyps enhance; allergic polyps do not.

Disadvantages

1. Nonionic contrast material is expensive.
2. The rare occurrence of a potentially fatal anaphylactic reaction to an intravenous contrast agent must be kept in mind.

In general, the use of intravenous contrast enhancement is limited to tumors, vascular lesions, and complicated paranasal sinus disease. Intravenous contrast medium is rarely administered in uncomplicated inflammatory and allergic sinusitis because of its expense.

ALTERNATIVE IMAGING MODALITIES

Tomography

Thin-section pluridirectional tomography is superior to plain radiographs in demonstrating bony lesions and soft tissue masses. Phantom artefacts can obscure small structures and small areas of significant disease. It should also be noted that the patient radiation dose for tomography is significantly higher than that for CT and that CT has a superior beam quality with less scatter.

The major advantage of tomography is the ease of availability, and there usually is no significant delay in scheduling a patient for tomograms. Tomograms can be done in the sagittal plane, which is not possible with CT scans. Both CT and magnetic resonance imaging (MRI) are the current imaging techniques of choice for head and neck lesions. The major advantage of CT over conventional tomography is its superior soft tissue resolution. Small opacities may be obscured by the blurring effect of conventional tomography. Minute details are well demonstrated by CT. Despite artefacts from dental fillings, the images are usually of diagnostic quality.

Magnetic Resonance Imaging

The principal indications for imaging with MRI are:

1. To assess the complications of inflammatory disease.
2. To assess the extent of malignant tumors. It is not uncommon for benign and malignant lesions to coexist, and malignant tumors can invoke an inflammatory response. MRI can define the margins of the tumor more precisely and thus prevent normal tissue from being irradiated.

T_1-weighted images assess anatomy; T_2-weighted images assess disease. Fluid-containing structures typically produce a brighter signal, whereas some of the malignant tumors produce a lower signal than normal structures do.

Advantages

An MRI scan can be performed in the axial, coronal, or sagittal plane and involves no radiation. Because bone does not cause any signal, artefacts seen at the base of the skull on CT are absent, resulting in superior soft tissue detail.

This makes MRI ideal for assessing any intraorbital or intracranial complications of paranasal sinus disease. Vascular structures are readily seen without use of intravenous contrast material.

Disadvantages

The major disadvantage of the MRI scan is that only a limited number of cases can be done because of the small number of scanners available. In addition, average time for a head scan with MRI is 30 to 45 minutes; the equivalent average CT scan time is approximately 15 minutes. The bones and the fine details of the lateral nasal wall are not well delineated on MRI. The MR scanner tends to be noisier and more confining than CT, and therefore claustrophobic patients are intolerant of this technique.

A head coil is used for paranasal sinus imaging. The future of MRI and fast scan techniques combined with paramagnetic contrast agents is promising for head and neck imaging.

Angiography

With the advent of CT and MRI scanning, angiography is now of limited value. It is still, however, useful for highly vascular tumors, especially angiofibroma. Angiography can be followed by embolization. Angiograms may also be indicated in cases of severe epistaxis.

Bone Scan

Radioisotope bone scanning with technetium 99m methylene diphosphate is useful for assessing metastatic spread of disease to bones. This technique is also useful in the assessment of some osteoblastic tumors.

Gallium M Scan

This is not a routine scan. When a tumor biopsy specimen is histologically a lymphoma, a gallium scan may identify the presence of systemic lymphoma. A gallium scan also has a role in assessment of abscesses and osteomyelitis.

4 Endoscopic and Radiologic Diagnosis

DIAGNOSTIC EVALUATION

A diagnostic nasal endoscopic examination is a routine component of the clinical evaluation of every patient with evident or suspected disease of the nose and paranasal sinuses in our institutions. The endoscope enables the examiner to recognize changes that may remain hidden from the naked eye and even from inspection with a microscope, thereby allowing diagnoses to be made, confirmed, expanded, or even revised, and the effects of topical and systemic therapy can be seen and evaluated.

The endoscopic examination also assists the physician in reaching a decision as to whether local or systemic medical therapy may be of value or whether surgical intervention is indicated. The indications for tomography or computed tomography (CT) are usually derived from a combination of the history and the endoscopic findings.

As a general rule, every patient scheduled for an endoscopic surgical procedure must have a CT scan or tomogram before surgery. Although CT increases the costs significantly, it is advisable, in our view, if only for medicolegal reasons (see Chapter 11).

INDICATIONS FOR TOMOGRAPHY

In a patient with a history of chronic, recurrent sinusitis over months or even years, in spite of repeated medical therapy, tomography should be performed when the diagnostic nasal endoscopic examination reveals changes in the lateral wall of the nose that can presumably be improved by surgery. Because a number of diseases of the lateral wall of the nose cannot be recognized and identified by endoscopy, we frequently perform tomography even when the endoscopic findings are normal, provided that the patient's history strongly suggests the presence of anterior ethmoidal disease.

Tomograms should always be done in those patients with a history of recurrent frontal or maxillary sinusitis that has been repeatedly treated by conservative means and when previous radiographs have confirmed the presence of a genuine sinus infection. Tomography in such cases will frequently identify the underlying predisposing anatomic variations or disease in the key sites, which can then be treated by a targeted, limited endoscopic procedure.

The time for performing the tomography or CT scan should be scheduled so that, if possible, it is done when the patient is relatively *symptom free*. Our intent is not to demonstrate diffuse mucous membrane swelling, the retention of secretions, or even to diagnose an empyema in one of the large paranasal sinuses but to document the underlying changes in the anterior ethmoidal sinus as clearly as possible. For this reason, it is important that chronic sinusitis be brought to an optimal condition by the use of appropriate local and medical therapy.

We have frequently observed in patients in whom tomograms were performed at the time of maximal symptoms and who subsequently came to surgery that even the most massive changes in the maxillary sinus (e.g., one that was completely opaque on the tomogram) had been dramatically improved in a short period by preoperative conservative medical therapy that reestablished ventilation and drainage. In some patients, maxillary sinus endoscopy often shows perfectly normal conditions, although 10 days earlier the tomograms showed marked polypoid swelling, cyst formation, or even total opacification of the maxillary sinus. These clinical observations suggest that not only are the mucosal changes in the maxillary sinus highly reversible and also that even though mucosal reactions may appear very rapidly, they can revert to normal with equal rapidity.

Tomograms and CT scans are also helpful for instructing and advising the patient. With the serial images, it is usually possible to explain the underlying pathophysiologic relationships and the need for surgery, even to a layperson. The tomograms can also be used to assist the surgeon in explaining the proposed surgical procedure to the patient. In addition, these images can be used to demonstrate the potential dangers of both the disease itself and those associated with the operative procedure by showing the proximity of the orbits, the base of the skull, and other structures.

PREPARATION FOR DIAGNOSTIC ENDOSCOPY

Before the nose is prepared for the diagnostic endoscopic examination, it should be examined by conventional anterior rhinoscopy to assess the state of the nose and the nasal mucous membranes before the application of a topical decongestant (Fig 4–1). The nasal mucosa is sprayed with a mixture of a topical anesthetic and a mild vasoconstrictor in equal parts. We use either 2% tetracaine (Pontocaine) and 0.1% xylometazoline (Otrivin) or 2% lidocaine (Xylocaine) and xylometazoline. A 5- to 10-minute period is then allowed for the vasoconstriction to take effect before commencing the examination.

The patient is placed in the supine position with the head turned toward the physician, who sits at the patient's right side. We prefer this position over the sitting one because the patient is more relaxed and the head, although movable, is well supported in two planes. This support minimizes the risk of mucosal injury from a sudden unintentional or reflex movement of the head. As an alternative, the patient can be examined in the sitting position, provided that the back of the head is supported by adjustable cups.

The following are basic instruments used for diagnostic endoscopy. Although a maxillary sinus trocar has been included in this list, it should be noted that maxillary sinus endoscopy is not a routine component of the diagnostic endoscopic procedure.

A

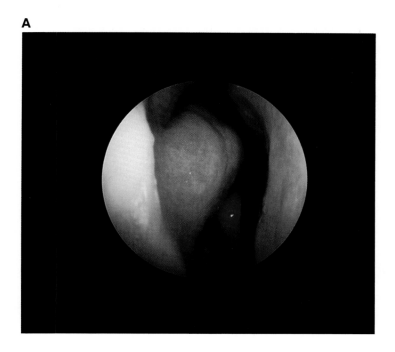

B

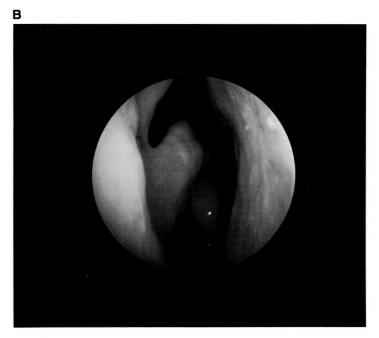

FIG 4–1.
A, inferior turbinate is filled with erectile tissue. In its normal state this erectile tissue is engorged, and consequently the inferior turbinate appears somewhat swollen. **B,** prior to endoscopic examination the inferior turbinate is placed in a state of vasoconstriction by application of a topical nasal decongestant. Note reduction in the size of the inferior turbinate. The anterior end of the middle turbinate can now be seen superoposterior to the anterior end of the inferior turbinate.

Nasal endoscopes
Essential
   0-degree lens, 4 mm with handle
   30-degree lens, 4 mm with handle
Useful additional lenses
   30-degree lens, 2.7 mm
   70-degree lens, 2.7 or 4 mm
Instruments
1 Freer elevator
1 flexible sound
1 assortment of suction tips
   (rigid and soft)
1 maxillary sinus trocar with sheath
1 biopsy forceps

TECHNIQUE OF DIAGNOSTIC ENDOSCOPY

The endoscopic examination of the nasal cavity and of the lateral wall of the nose is usually accomplished in three steps:

1. Inspection of the nasal vestibule, the nasopharynx, and the inferior nasal meatus
2. Examination of the sphenoethmoidal recess and the superior nasal meatus
3. Examination of the middle meatus

The best endoscopes for the routine diagnostic nasal endoscopic examination are either the 0-degree, wide-angle 4-mm diameter endoscope or the 30-degree, 4-mm diameter endoscope. When the nasal passages are very narrow, the narrower 2.7-mm diameter endoscopes with either a 30- or 70-degree lens angle may be required.

Before use, the lens should be dipped briefly into an antifogging solution (e.g., Ultrastop). It is important that the antifogging solution not be wiped off the lens before the endoscope is introduced into the nose, because a thin film of the antifog solution must remain on the lens to assure freedom from fogging. Before starting the examination, the physician and the patient should agree on a signal that the patient can give if a sneeze or a cough is coming on. This will allow the examiner to quickly withdraw the endoscope and any other instruments from the nose so that injuries from involuntary sneezing and coughing can be avoided.

When an endoscope is introduced into the nose it is important not to injure the mucous membrane, and every effort should be made by the examiner to keep the lens away from the nasal mucous membrane throughout the entire procedure.

The endoscopic examination of the nose should be performed in a systematic manner.

Inspection of Nasal Vestibule, Nasopharynx, and Inferior Nasal Meatus

The first look provides a general survey and orientation within the nose. The examiner should first look in the direction of the middle meatus without actually

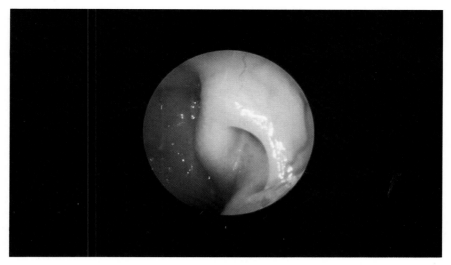

FIG 4–2.
Eustachian tube ostium. Note how well the ostium of the eustachian tube and the surrounding torus tubarius can be seen with the endoscope.

approaching it too closely. This will provide an excellent overview of the nose, and allows identification of gross anatomic or pathologic abnormalities. The appearance, color, engorgement, and presence or absence of pathologic secretions on the mucous membranes can be assessed and the width of the nasal cavity determined.

Septal deviations, ridges, and spurs can also be evaluated as to their size and extent. The foamy secretions that are frequently encountered in the narrow spaces in the nose after the application of a local anesthetic spray should be removed with an aspirator introduced parallel to the endoscope. An attempt is then made to reach the nasopharynx through the nasal cavity with the endoscope. Depending on the anatomic configuration, this can usually be accomplished without difficulty by advancing the endoscope medial to the inferior turbinate. If there is not enough room between the inferior turbinate and the septum, the endoscope is advanced along the floor of the inferior meatus. The ostium of the eustachian tube can be used as a landmark in the nasopharynx (Fig 4–2). The function of the torus tubarius can be observed when the patient swallows on command. At this point, abnormalities in the transportation of secretions may be observed (e.g., pathologic secretions) that lie centrally over the tube or that remain attached in Rosenmueller's fossa. When the 30-degree endoscope is used, a slight medial rotation of the endoscope along its long axis allows inspection of the posterior wall of the nasopharynx and of the roof of the palate.

In the nasopharynx, the examiner can assess the shape and size and the presence or absence of inflammation of the adenoids or see the scars where this tissue was removed. Occasionally a small slit or a round opening can be seen that enters into a small depression or into a superiorly directed passage. This is the remnant of a Rathke pouch. At times a drop of viscous secretion can be seen in a Rathke pocket. If the endoscope is then rotated further medially, the examiner can see the ostium of the eustachian tube on the opposite side.

In this manner the examiner can inspect the entire nasopharynx with the 30-degree lens. This is especially useful when a marked septal deviation or other pathologic condition makes it impossible to introduce the endoscope through the other side of the nose. The endoscope can now be rotated a full 360 degrees around its longitudinal axis, and the posterior aspect of the uvula and the nasal surface of the palate inspected. Pulling the endoscope back a few millimeters and rotating it fully permits evaluation of the margins of the choana and the posterior end of the turbinates.

The examiner should keep in mind during the endoscopic examination of the nasopharynx that the wide-angle effect of the lens makes all curved surfaces appear much flatter in the frontal view. Thus those abnormalities that are raised *above the level of the mucous membranes* and that show no alteration in color or structure may be overlooked. It is therefore essential for a complete examination of the nasopharynx that this area also be inspected from the oropharynx with either a mirror or a 90-degree endoscope. The tangential view over the surface of the nasopharyngeal mucous membranes obtained with these techniques allows discrete elevations to be recognized with a greater degree of accuracy.

If the examiner now pulls the endoscope back, a look under the inferior turbinate can be attempted. The opening of the nasolacrimal duct (Hasner's valve) may be observed within a few millimeters of the highest point of the roof of the inferior nasal meatus, at the transition to the lateral wall (Fig 4–3). The opening of the nasolacrimal duct into the inferior meatus may be round, although it may have almost any form, including that of an almost invisible slit hidden behind a fold of mucosa. The patency of the nasolacrimal duct can be assessed by instilling a drop of fluorescein into the conjunctival sac and observing the emergence of the dye in the inferior nasal meatus. The easiest way to identify the opening of the nasolacrimal duct is to put light finger pressure on the lacrimal sac at the medial angle of the eyelid. This pressure usually expresses a few tears from the opening of the nasolacrimal duct, which can be easily seen with the endoscope.

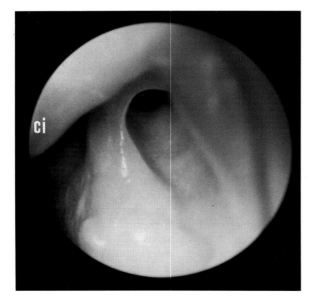

FIG 4–3.
Well-developed Hasner's valve (ostium of the nasolacrimal duct) in a left inferior meatus. *ci* = inferior turbinate.

Depending on the shape of the inferior turbinate, entry into the inferior nasal meatus may be difficult, particularly if the horizontal part of the turbinate is small and the vertical part reaches down almost to the floor of the meatus or is curled up laterally. Careful elevation of the free margin of the inferior turbinate with a Freer elevator, combined if necessary with the use of a thinner 2.7-mm diameter nasal endoscope, usually permits a reasonable view in these cases.

Examination of Sphenoethmoidal Recess and Superior Nasal Meatus

In the second step of the diagnostic nasal examination, the endoscope is directed medial to the middle turbinate in the direction of the nasopharynx and the end of the middle turbinate is identified. Above this, the view should be directed superiorly toward the sphenoethmoidal recess. Laterally the inferior free margin of the superior turbinate can be seen. The superior nasal meatus and the cells of the posterior ethmoid that open into the superior meatus opening are located below the superior turbinate. Occasionally there may be a vestigial or even a well-developed supreme (fourth) turbinate, under which openings of the posterior ethmoidal cells can also be found.

The posterior wall of the sphenoethmoidal recess is formed by the anterior surface of the sphenoid bone. Here the oval or slitlike ostium of the sphenoid sinus can usually be found in the medial part of the posterior wall of the sphenoethmoidal recess near the posterior insertion of the nasal septum. If the passage is very narrow or there is an evident pathologic condition, it may be difficult to positively identify the ostium of the sphenoidal sinus with the endoscope. If the sphenoidal sinus is diseased, the presence of abnormal secretions on the anterior surface of the sphenoid may indicate the location of the ostium of the sphenoidal sinus (Fig 4–4).

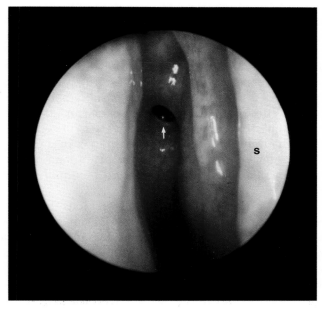

FIG 4–4.
After the secretions were aspirated, a narrowed sphenoid sinus ostium can be seen (*arrow*). *s* = nasal septum.

Examination of Middle Meatus

The third step in the diagnostic nasal examination consists of exploration of the middle meatus and, within it, the adjacent lateral nasal wall. This is accomplished by advancing the 30-degree endoscope to the entrance to the middle meatus and identifying the structures in this area. Viewing from the front, the examiner can usually readily see the head of the middle turbinate, the uncinate process, and depending on the presence of pathologic changes, parts of the ethmoid bulla (Fig 4–5). Occasionally it is possible to enter the middle meatus directly from in front with the endoscope and view the inferior and superior hiatus semilunaris, the sinus of the turbinate, and even the frontal recess. If the superior hiatus semilunaris is wide, it may be possible to look into the lateral sinus and see the ridge of the anterior ethmoidal artery running along the roof of the ethmoid (Fig 4–6).

When it is impossible to enter the middle meatus with the endoscope from the anterior, the following options are available. It may be possible to gently displace the middle turbinate medially (as far as its elasticity permits) with a Freer elevator or a thin aspirator. In doing this, the examiner should take care not to fracture the middle turbinate. The middle meatus can also be examined through a trocar sheath, as described by Messerklinger. The endoscope is placed into the trocar sheath, which is then introduced into the nose. The flat lip of the trocar sheath frequently can be slipped underneath the middle turbinate, and through careful rotatory movements advanced into the middle meatus. The scope is advanced through the sheath and an unobstructed view of the middle meatus obtained.

Because the middle meatus is usually wider at the back than in the front, the technique that we most use frequently in this situation is to inspect the middle meatus with the endoscope from the back. The 30-degree scope is introduced past the middle turbinate toward the back, and then is rotated laterally and superiorly under the free margin of the turbinate (see Fig 8–12). This maneuver usually allows the endoscope to be slipped into the most posterior portion of the middle meatus. Careful, slow retraction of the endoscope then permits inspection of the middle meatus from the rear forward. The first structure seen is the horizontal part of the middle turbinate (i.e., posterior third of the basal lamella), which here forms the roof of the middle meatus and curves upward behind the ethmoidal bulla as the basal lamella to separate the anterior and posterior ethmoidal sinuses. Farther forward, the bulge of the ethmoidal bulla can be seen. Between the medial surface of the ethmoidal bulla and the vertical part of the middle turbinate, one can look into the sinus of the turbinate and farther anteriorly into the superior semilunar hiatus (when present), which opens into the lateral sinus above and eventually passes behind the ethmoidal bulla.

A slight rotation of the 30-degree lens laterally will bring the hiatus semilunaris into view between the anterior surface of the bulla and the free posterior margin of the uncinate process. Anatomic conditions permitting, the endoscope can be directed slightly upward, so that the hiatus semilunaris can be followed and the frontal recess inspected (see Fig 4–6). The ostia and openings of the cells and spaces visible here depend on the status of the uncinate process and the lamella of the bulla.

The natural ostium of the maxillary sinus is only rarely visible from the middle meatus. Occasionally a direct view into the maxillary sinus is possible

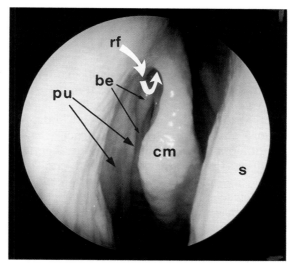

FIG 4–5.
View into a normal right middle meatus. The uncinate process and its posterior free edge, and the anterior surface of the ethmoidal bulla can be seen. The *white arrows* indicate the path into the frontal recess behind the insertion of the middle turbinate. *rf* = frontal recess; *be* = ethmoidal bulla; *pu* = uncinate process; *cm* = middle turbinate; *s* = nasal septum.

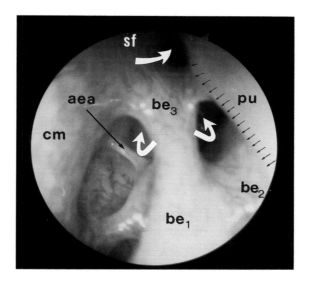

FIG 4–6.
View into a left frontal recess through a 30-degree, wide-angle endoscope. The anterior wall of the bulla ethmoidalis passes superiorly into a bulla lamella. The bulla lamella is attached medially to the insertion of the middle turbinate and superiorly to the skull, although not along its entire length. There is a marked lateral sinus between the bulla itself and the roof of the ethmoid. The lateral sinus opens medially and laterally to the bulla lamella (*angled arrows*). The bony channel of the anterior ethmoidal artery can be seen clearly. Superiorly, the frontal recess narrows toward the ostium of the frontal sinus (arrow). The *thin arrows* point to the free posterior margin of the uncinate process. be_1 = anterior wall of the bulla ethmoidalis; be_2 = insertion of the bulla ethmoidalis onto the lamina papyracea; be_3 = bulla lamella; *cm* = middle turbinate; *aea* = anterior ethmoidal artery; *sf* = frontal sinus; *pu* = uncinate process.

through an accessory ostium in the anterior or posterior nasal fontanelles. It is sometimes possible to see the maxillary ostium in the depths of the ethmoidal infundibulum through a wide hiatus semilunaris from the back with a 70-degree lens.

Because the 70-degree lens does not permit forward vision and consequently there is a danger of injury to the nasal mucous membranes when the scope is advanced, we use the following technique.

A trocar sheath is slipped over a 0- or 30-degree endoscope and introduced into the nose. Under direct vision, the trocar sheath is brought into the position to be examined and fixed while the guide scope is removed and the 70-degree lens introduced through the trocar sheath and advanced to the end of the trocar sheath. The area of interest can then be examined. With this technique, the 70-degree telescope can be inserted without coming into contact with the mucous membranes.

Because this procedure exerts greater pressure on the middle turbinate and nasal septum, it may be necessary to use nasal pledgets, in addition to the topical spray, to achieve more complete anesthesia. We use small cotton applicators that have been dipped in a mixture of 2% tetracaine (Pontocaine) and 1:1,000 epinephrine (4–5:1). The excess anesthetic solution is squeezed out; then the cotton applicators are placed into and around the middle meatus and left there for 5 to 10 minutes. Following this, contact with the trocar sleeve and endoscope or other instruments should no longer be painful.

This anesthetic technique is also useful in those cases in which a biopsy is indicated. When the nasopharynx is to be biopsied and the nasal cavities are narrow, we will introduce the endoscope through one side of the nose and the biopsy forceps through the opposite side.

If diagnostic endoscopy is indicated in a young child, the procedure should be performed with the child under sedation or general anesthesia, depending on the patient's ability to cooperate.

ENDOSCOPIC AND RADIOLOGIC APPEARANCE OF COMMON ABNORMALITIES OF NASAL CAVITY AND PARANASAL SINUSES

Nasal Septal Deviations

Severe deviation of the entire nasal septum or of a portion of the septum may cause not only obstructed nasal breathing but also disease within the lateral nasal wall and consequently within the paranasal sinuses. This is especially true if the septal deviation forces the middle turbinate laterally and narrows the entrance into the middle meatus.

Septal ridges and spurs can be the cause of severe headaches and other functional disturbances, especially if they come into intimate contact with the turbinates or other areas of the lateral wall of the nose. Septal ridges and spurs can regularly surround the middle turbinate, and on occasion may project far into the middle meatus, significantly affecting nasal function and predisposing to recurrent sinus infections.

Clinical experience shows, however, that many patients with massive septal deviation, ridges, or spurs may have no symptoms or only minimal complaints attributable to these changes. They may instead have symptoms on the opposite side (i.e., on the side with the wider nasal passage). For this reason, we have become reluctant to correct a septal deviation except in extreme cases, and then only when there is a clear connection between the deviation of the nasal septum and the clinical symptoms (Fig 4–7). Our experience has shown that most patients can be rendered symptom free after correction of the ethmoid problems without having the (occasionally severe) nasal septal deviation corrected at the same time. We therefore do not support the dictum that every endonasal surgical procedure on the paranasal sinuses be preceded by the correction of any preexisting deviation of the nasal septum.

Our procedure in cases of documented ethmoidal sinus disease and nasal septal deviations is therefore as follows.

If there is enough room to pass both the 4-mm endoscope and the other necessary surgical instruments beyond the septal deviation into the affected middle meatus, we first correct the ethmoidal problems surgically. The surgical procedure may be more difficult under these circumstances, and it is even more important to proceed as atraumatically as possible. Injuries to the mucous

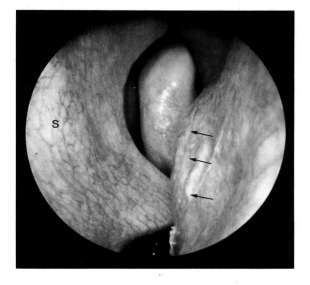

FIG 4–7.
The septal ridge that extends both anterior and inferior to the left middle meatus terminates in a huge septal spur that impinges on the inferior turbinate. The mucosa of the inferior turbinate is hyperplastic in this area (*arrows*). The septal spur did not obstruct access to the middle meatus but was resected because of its impingement on the middle turbinate. *s* = septum.

membranes in the middle meatus, septum, or lateral nasal wall must be avoided. We have found it advantageous in such cases not to attempt to advance the endoscope as close to the middle meatus as possible but only close enough to get a good view of the middle meatus.

Only when the deviation is so severe that the endoscope and the instruments cannot be introduced through the narrowed area do we perform a septoplasty as the first procedure, and then we wait a few weeks until the nose has fully recovered. If the sinus complaints persist unchanged after correction of the nasal septal deviation and a repeat diagnostic endoscopy still shows findings characteristic of ethmoid disease, the ethmoidal problems are corrected endoscopically at a second procedure. The only exception is in the patient with severe nasal polyps and a significantly obstructing nasal septal deviation. In this situation we perform both procedures at the same time. Since we have adopted this philosophy, the need for septoplasty in our patients has decreased, and it is currently well below 10% of all paranasal sinus procedures.

Septal ridges or spurs may project into the uncinate process or hiatus semilunaris and cause additional problems. Smaller septal ridges and spurs that seem to be part of the disease process or that interfere with direct surgical access to the middle meatus can be resected in isolation as part of the endoscopic procedure without performing a complete septoplasty. The mucosa surrounding the spur is injected with local anesthetic and incised, and the spur is dissected free. In most cases these isolated spurs can be easily removed with a chisel or a conchotome.

Septal Tubercle

The septal tubercle, or swell body, consists of a localized submucosal area of erectile tissue in the anterior portion of the nasal septum. At first glance, this convexly elevated septal mucosa may appear to be a septal deviation. If the examiner looks into the opposite nasal cavity, a similar "deviation" will be seen. Gentle compression over this area with the endoscope or aspiration will confirm the presence of erectile tissue as the "deviation" collapses under pressure (Fig 4–8).

ANATOMIC VARIATIONS OF MIDDLE TURBINATE

Concha Bullosa

Pneumatization of the middle turbinate, and less commonly of the superior turbinate, can be clinically significant, and is known as a concha bullosa. Concha bullosa usually occurs bilaterally; however, the degree of pneumatization may be variable not only from patient to patient but also from one side to the other in a given patient. The pneumatized area may be so small that it appears on only one section of the tomogram or CT scan. In contrast, the degree of pneumatization may be so severe that both middle turbinates, expanded like balloons, come into intimate and extensive contact with large areas of the septum and with the entire lateral wall (Fig 4–9). In rare cases, a massive

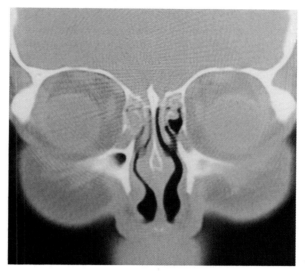

FIG 4–8.
Septal tubercle (nasal septal swell body). Symmetric soft tissue swelling on either side of the middle of the nasal septum in this coronal CT scan is an engorged nasal septal tubercle.

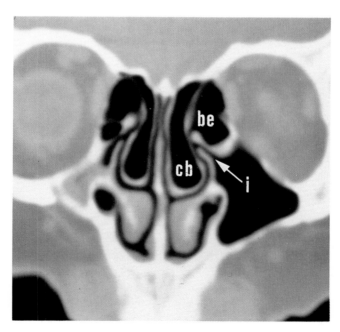

FIG 4–9.
In this patient, the concha bullosa was pneumatized from the frontal recess and the lateral sinus. *be* = bulla ethmoidalis; *cb* = concha bullosa; *i* = infundibulum.

concha bullosa can completely obstruct the nasal cavity (Fig 4–10).

Large differences in the degree of pneumatization between both sides are found most commonly in those patients who also have marked deviation of the nasal septum. Pneumatization of the middle turbinate may originate from a variety of sites. In our experience, the most common site of origin is the frontal recess (see Fig 4–9). Pneumatization may also originate from the agger nasi, which is itself usually pneumatized from the frontal recess or even from the lateral sinus. Pneumatization may come directly from the middle meatus. In some patients the superior meatus may intrude into the middle turbinate to such degree that extensive pneumatization results. This type of concha bullosa was called an "interlamellar cell" by Grünwald.

In most cases a concha bullosa contains only a single air cell, although occasionally two, and very rarely three, air cells are encountered. These multiple air cells are usually located one behind the other. In these cases, pneumatization does not necessarily originate from a single site. The anterior cell is usually pneumatized from the frontal recess, and the posterior cell directly from the middle meatus. Although these multiple cells may communicate, in most cases they are completely sealed off from each other.

The ventilation of the air cells within a concha bullosa comes from the same area from which the pneumatization arose. Mucociliary transport is also directed in the same direction. Thus the secretions from a concha bullosa pneumatized from the frontal recess are transported to the frontal recess, where they join the regular transportation pathway to the nasopharynx (see Chapter 1).

This relationship indicates a reciprocal susceptibility whereby it is possible for disease in a frontal recess to spread into its connected concha bullosa. Conversely, disease may spread from an infected turbinate cell to other connected areas of the ethmoidal sinus.

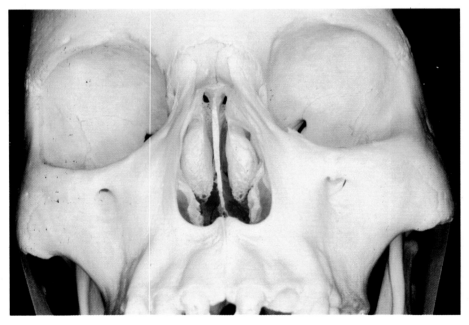

FIG 4–10.
Bilateral large concha bullosa. Massive symmetric thickening of the middle turbinates seen in the nasal cavity of this skull are extremely large concha bullosa.

The interior of a concha bullosa can be affected by any of the disease processes that may affect any paranasal sinus. These may range from simple edema of the mucosal lining as part of a disease of the frontal recess, to the formation of a single or multiple polyps, the retention of secretions with the radiologic evidence of an air fluid level, empyemas, the accumulation of amorphous, inspissated secretions, the formation of a mucocele or even of a pyocele, and finally to fungal infections, with accumulation of mycotic concretions in the lumen of the turbinate itself.

In those patients who have extensive, diffuse, long-standing nasal polyposis, the recognition of a concha bullosa on a conventional tomogram may be very difficult, particularly in the older patient, in whom the thin bony lamellae may be decalcified or thinned by the pressure exerted by the polyps or largely destroyed by the inflammatory process. In such cases, the definite diagnosis of a diseased concha bullosa may be made only at surgery, by making an exploratory incision through the anterior wall of the middle turbinate with a curved blade.

A concha bullosa alone is not necessarily a pathologic finding. However, even small pneumatizations, if combined with other anatomic abnormalities such as a medially bent uncinate process or an enlarged ethmoidal bulla, may produce significant narrowing of the anterior and middle portions of the middle meatus. Large contact surfaces may appear that predispose to repeated, and later to persistent local complaints that may spread to involve the adjacent areas. If the pneumatization is extensive, a large concha bullosa may cause significant problems by its size alone (e.g., marked nasal obstruction or blocked nasal respiration; (see Figs 4–9 and 4–10). The disturbance of the transportation of secretions that results from such extensive areas of mucosal contact may well be the cause of the unpleasant postnasal drip of which many patients with large concha bullosa so frequently complain.

In some patients, the outward bulging of the lateral lamella of a concha bullosa appears to push against the lateral wall of the nose to such extent that it displaces the uncinate process laterally. This may produce narrowing or even complete blockage of the hiatus semilunaris and of the ethmoidal infundibulum. A nondiseased concha bullosa can cause critical narrowing in the anterior ethmoidal sinus. In these cases, only a minimal amount of mucosal swelling (e.g., as the result of the normal nasal cycle, a sudden change in temperature, minor infection, or other slight irritation) may partially or completely close this narrow cleft, producing all of the potentially deleterious consequences for the anterior ethmoidal and the larger paranasal sinuses.

The concha bullosa is a classic example of the potential of an anatomic variant to predispose to sinus disease. A concha bullosa by itself does not represent a disease state per se, but it predisposes under certain conditions to sinus infections more readily and more frequently. Even relatively minor stimuli that in a person without a concha bullosa would cause only a temporary feeling of nasal stuffiness, somewhat increased secretions, or a minor rhinitis may in patients with a concha bullosa cause sufficient mucosal swelling to produce complete obstruction of the key sites in the ethmoidal sinus, thereby leading to the appearance or persistence of major symptoms.

We have frequently observed this sequence of events in patients with hay fever or other inhalational allergies. The slight mucosal swelling triggered by an allergic reaction is sufficient to cause severe symptoms. In these cases, surgical resection of the concha bullosa should be considered as adjuvant therapy, which usually results in a marked improvement of their nasal symptoms. This facilitates the antiallergic or hyposensitization therapy and allows the use of lower doses or fewer medications.

The concha bullosa also illustrates the significant role that mucosal contact areas play in the formation of nasal polyps. Frequently the mucosal contact areas are the first to show a circumscribed area of edema that may later serve as the base for extensive polyp formation (Fig 4–11).

Endoscopically a concha bullosa usually manifests as an enlarged or widened head or body of the middle turbinate that may come into contact medially with the nasal septum and that bulges laterally widely into the lateral wall of the nose, thereby making inspection of the middle meatus impossible. The typical appearance of a concha bullosa is shown in (see Figs 4–10 and 4–11).

It should be emphasized that a concha bullosa cannot always be identified with the nasal endoscope. The wide angle of the endoscope tends to make objects look smaller than they really are. What appears in the endoscope as a relatively normal middle turbinate often appears to be much larger when examined directly, as with a nasal speculum. Occasionally, relatively innocuous appearing middle turbinates may contain extensive pneumatization, and conversely, not every widened head of a middle turbinate is pneumatized.

When there are extensive pathologic conditions within the nose, endoscopic diagnosis may be extremely difficult, and the diagnosis will have to be made with conventional tomography or CT, although even these techniques can have their limitations.

Pneumatization of the superior turbinate is extremely rare, and only a few cases have been reported in which the symptoms of a superior turbinate concha bullosa were sufficiently severe to require surgical correction. In these rare cases the pneumatization of the superior turbinates was bilateral and forced the turbinates so far anterior between the septum and the middle turbinate that headaches and a loss of olfactory sensation resulted.

In addition to a concha bullosa, the middle turbinate may have other significant anatomic variations that can narrow the middle meatus and produce mucosal contact sites.

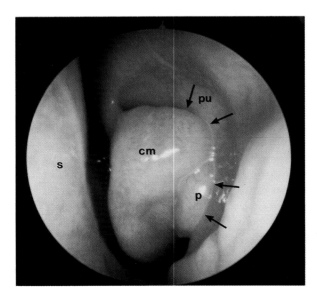

FIG 4–11.
Concha bullosa of the left middle turbinate. The turbinate is in close contact (*arrows*) with the lateral wall of the nose in the area of the uncinate process. Polypoid mucosa spills out around the area of contact. The head of the concha bullosa shows some edematous changes. *s* = nasal septum; *cm* = middle turbinate; *pu* = uncinate process; *p* = polyp.

Enlarged and Anterior Extending Middle Turbinates

A distended head of the middle turbinate is not always caused by abnormalities of the mucous membranes. L- or T-shaped underlying bony lamellae of the turbinate are the usual cause of the triangular-appearing middle turbinate.

The vertical bony lamella of the middle turbinate can assume a variety of curvatures. The head of the middle turbinate may have normal medial convexity, whereas in its posterior two thirds it may instead have a significant paradoxical bend (laterally directed convexity). This is most frequently seen when the anterior third of the turbinate contains a concha bullosa.

It is important to remember during surgery that the shape and contour of the head of the middle turbinate are not reliable topographic landmarks (see Chapter 2). Normally the head of the middle turbinate extends only a few millimeters anterior to its attachment on the lateral nasal wall. The anterior surface of the head of the middle turbinate usually follows in its contours the projection of the attachment of the uncinate process along the lateral nasal wall. There are, however, frequent variations in which the head of the middle turbinate extends beyond its attachment by more than 1 cm, thereby overlapping the uncinate process by a considerable margin and sometimes to such extent that it even overlies a portion of the agger nasi.

These variations of the head of the turbinate must be considered when the attachment of the uncinate process must be identified before the infundibulum is opened.

Paradoxically Bent Middle Turbinate

In the so-called paradoxically bent middle turbinate, the turbinate is curved laterally; that is, the concavity of the turbinate points toward the septum and its convexity toward the lateral wall (Fig 4–12). Paradoxically bent middle turbinates usually occur bilaterally.

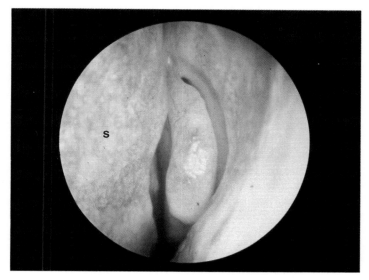

FIG 4–12.
Minimally bent paradoxical left middle turbinate. The patient is in a symptom-free interval. *s* = nasal septum.

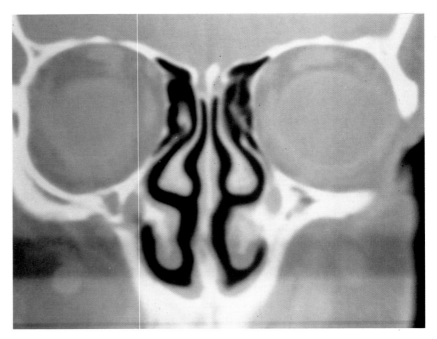

FIG 4–13.
Marked, bilateral, paradoxically bent middle turbinates. The relative constriction of the middle meatus and particularly of the ethmoidal infundibulum is clearly visible.

A paradoxically bent middle turbinate by itself is not a pathologic finding, although in some cases the paradoxic curvature may be quite pronounced and thereby cause significant narrowing of the entrance to the middle meatus. In this instance, a paradoxically bent middle turbinate may be combined with another anatomic variation to produce severe narrowing of the entrance to the middle meatus with extensive areas of mucosal contact (see Fig 4–12). The most important combination is with a medially bent uncinate process. Severe paradoxically bent middle turbinates can, on occasion, make endoscopic surgical manipulations on the ethmoidal sinus very difficult (Fig 4–13), and in rare instances a limited resection of the anterior end of the middle turbinate may be necessary to gain access to the middle meatus for an endoscopic procedure.

A normally curved middle turbinate may occasionally be so tightly rolled up laterally that it may mimic a concha bullosa on the x-ray image. The free margin of such a middle turbinate may be curved so far laterally that it envelops the middle meatus and makes introduction of an endoscope almost impossible. The space under the concavity of such a middle turbinate, which is frequently filled by a large ethmoidal bulla, has been called a sinus conchae or turbinate sinus.

ABNORMALITIES OF UNCINATE PROCESS

The uncinate process may show a large number of anatomic variations. Normally the uncinate process extends from its sickle-shaped attachment on the lateral wall of the nose and the inferior turbinate posteriorly and medially to its posterior free margin, so that only a 1- to 3-mm wide fissure, the hiatus semilunaris, remains between the posterior free border of the uncinate process and the anterior surface of the ethmoidal bulla. The distance between the posterior free margin of the uncinate process and the lamina papyracea varies between 1.5 and 5 mm.

Medially Bent Uncinate Process

The most common and pathologically significant variation of the uncinate process is a marked medial curvature or bend of the uncinate process. This medial bending may involve the entire uncinate process or only certain portions of it, so that at times the uncinate process appears like a twisted band. The medial curvature can be so marked that its free edge and even its entire medial surface come into contact with the lateral surface of the middle turbinate.

The uncinate process can be bent medially and folded anteriorly so far that it protrudes anteriorly and inferiorly into the middle meatus, like the curled brim of a hat (Fig 4–14). This may give the impression that two middle

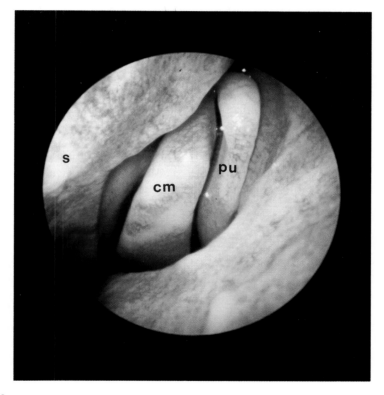

FIG 4–14.
"Doubled" middle turbinate. The uncinate process on the left side is bent medially anteriorly and inferiorly so that it protrudes from the middle meatus, parallel to the middle turbinate. It thus appeared as though there were a second middle turbinate. s = septum; *cm* = middle turbinate; *pu* = uncinate process.

turbinates are present. Kaufmann called this abnormality a reduplication of the middle turbinate.

A markedly medially bent or folded uncinate process, with a corresponding area of extensive contact with the middle turbinate, is one of the most frequent pathologic findings in those patients with a history of recurrent sinus infections.

In its projection superiorly, the uncinate process may bend laterally and insert onto the lamina papyracea, thereby closing off blindly the ethmoidal infundibulum superiorly and forming a terminal recess (see Fig 2–15). When this happens, the secretions from the frontal recess are carried past the ethmoidal infundibulum medially and arrive inferiorly at the hiatus semilunaris. Through accessory ostia in the fontanelles, these secretions may even be transported into the maxillary sinus.

On occasion the uncinate process may extend upward to reach the base of the skull. When this happens, the frontal recess will open inferiorly, directly into the ethmoidal infundibulum. The superior portion of the uncinate process may also be twisted medially and undergo a bony fusion with the attachment of the middle turbinate or even with parts of the head of the turbinate. In extreme cases, this may produce an almost frontally oriented bony plate, which can narrow the entrance to the middle meatus and the frontal recess anteriorly, much like a postoperative adhesion.

Laterally Bent Uncinate Process

The uncinate process may also be bent laterally, either along its entire length or in only one portion. This lateral displacement of the uncinate process can narrow the ethmoid infundibulum, especially when the uncinate process inserts far laterally on the inferior turbinate.

In the radiologic assessment of the uncinate process in coronal sections, its anatomic course must always be kept in mind. As a result of its arc-shaped course, the most anterior coronal sections will show the uncinate process at its widest. In the middle third of its course, the uncinate process appears to lie immediately adjacent to the posterior wall of the nasolacrimal duct. In the more posterior sections it appears increasingly narrower because of its arc from anterosuperior to posteroinferior.

Elongated and Enlarged Uncinate Processes

The uncinate process may extend too far posteriorly. With this increased posterior extension, the uncinate process may impinge its free posterior margin onto the ethmoidal bulla, thereby significantly narrowing the hiatus semilunaris. The same result can be achieved if the uncinate process overlaps the bulla medially and posteriorly. When combined with other anatomic variations, such as a paradoxically curved middle turbinate, a concha bullosa, or an excessively pneumatized ethmoidal bulla, such abnormalities of the uncinate process may produce significant functional blockade of the narrow spaces of the anterior ethmoidal sinus and of the related frontal and maxillary sinuses.

The strength of this small bony plate varies enormously. In cases of chronic polyposis or other inflammatory diseases, its bony plate may become so demineralized that it becomes invisible on radiographs, and may even defy identification at surgery.

Secondary Changes in Uncinate Process

Because the uncinate process forms the bony medial wall of the ethmoidal infundibulum, any pathologic changes in the uncinate process or in its medial mucosal covering are important indicators of an inflammatory process or disease within the infundibulum itself. Changes in the mucous membrane covering the medial surface of the uncinate process suggest changes in the infundibulum, the frontal recess, and the adjacent areas of the anterior ethmoid. Frequently these changes consist of discrete, circumscribed mucosal swellings at the site of contact. Such extensive contact between the uncinate process and the middle turbinate and also the ethmoidal bulla can be diagnosed in many cases by carefully displacing the middle turbinate medially with a Freer elevator.

Other times these alterations may consist of polypoid changes. These polyps, which originate from the free margin of the uncinate process or from within the infundibulum proper, may protrude around the free edge of the uncinate process into the nasal cavity. Frequently the entire medial wall of the infundibulum bulges medially, indicating the presence of a significant pathologic process in the anterior ethmoid. The changes may consist of chronic edema, and in acute exacerbations perforations may develop in the uncinate process through which pus or other abnormal secretions may come pouring forth.

The mucosa over the posterior margin and on the lateral surface of the uncinate process (medial wall of the ethmoidal infundibulum) appears to be particularly sensitive to inflammatory stimuli, and responds readily with engorgement and polyp formation. We have frequently observed in patients with extensive nasal polyps that resection of the uncinate process usually removes the most anterior large polyps, indicating that these polyps arose from the uncinate process and from the ethmoidal infundibulum. This clinical observation is the reason why in these patients we try to identify and resect the uncinate process first and not just remove the polyps that seem to be obstructing the passage toward it. This technique is much less bloody and provides better exposure, thereby permitting a tissue-sparing, goal-oriented operation.

Pneumatization of Uncinate Process

The uncinate process may in rare cases be pneumatized. When the uncinate process is pneumatized, the additional space occupied by this widened structure causes further narrowing of the already narrow spaces of the ethmoidal infundibulum and creates new areas of mucosal contact.

ACCESSORY MAXILLARY SINUS OSTIA

The natural ostium of the maxillary sinus can almost never be seen directly from the middle meatus, because it is hidden behind the uncinate process in the depths of the posterior third of the ethmoidal infundibulum. In more than 25% of patients, "holes," or ostia, can be found in the lateral nasal wall leading into the maxillary sinus. These holes may be located both anteriorly and posteriorly, directly below the posterior third of the uncinate process. These are accessory maxillary sinus ostia through the anterior and posterior nasal fontanelles (see Figs 2–3 and 4–15) and not the natural ostium of the maxillary sinus. It is not unusual to find secretions moving through the accessory ostia into the maxillary sinus. These secretions then leave the maxillary sinus through its natural ostium, passing through the ethmoidal infundibulum, where they may mingle with the secretions carried toward the maxillary sinus and thus proceed in a circle. This mechanism provides a route along which pathogens may be carried into the maxillary sinus when its natural ostium is closed (see Chapter 1).

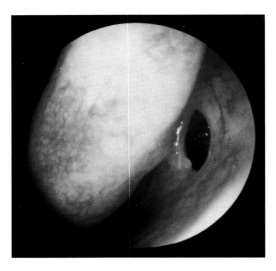

FIG 4–15.
This patient has a large accessory maxillary sinus ostium.

ETHMOIDAL BULLA

The ethmoidal bulla (bulla ethmoidalis) is usually the largest, most constant, and easily identifiable air cell of the anterior ethmoid. It rests laterally on the lamina papyracea, although its other relationships are highly variable. The bulla can extend superiorly to the roof of the ethmoid and posteriorly to the basal lamella of the middle turbinate. Depending on the development of a lateral sinus or other anterior ethmoidal cells, the bulla may lose contact with the roof of the ethmoid and also with the basal lamella (see Chapter 2). Although the ethmoidal bulla may become independently diseased, clinical experience shows that most diseases of the bulla originate more frequently at its contact sites with other structures rather than from the interior of the bulla.

Enlarged Ethmoidal Bulla

The extent of pneumatization of the ethmoidal bulla is variable, ranging from no pneumatization at all to extensive pneumatization, where the bulla extends far anteriorly under the middle turbinate (Fig 4–16). An excessively pneumatized bulla may expand anteriorly, coming into intimate contact with the posterior free margin of the uncinate process, thereby narrowing or partially blocking the hiatus semilunaris. The bulla may also expand medially beyond the hiatus semilunaris and block it. Finally, the pneumatization can extend so far anteriorly that the bulla forces its way between the uncinate process and the head of the middle turbinate (Fig 4–17). When examined from anteriorly, this

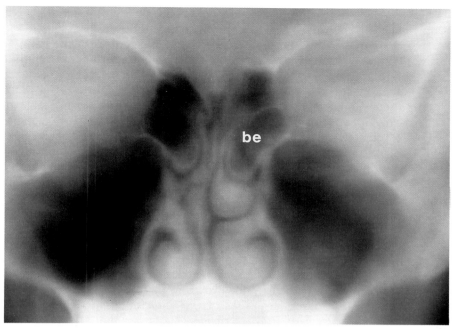

FIG 4–16.
This scan shows bilateral large ethmoidal bullae. Even though the bullar air cells are healthy in this case, such extensive pneumatization can be the cause of numerous symptoms. *be* = bulla ethmoidalis.

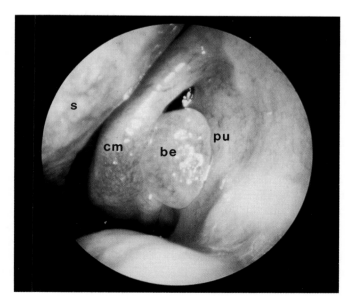

FIG 4–17.
Note the large bulla herniating from the middle meatus. Extensive pneumatization has caused the bulla to extend anteriorly. The mucous membrane shows polypoid changes. *s* = septum; *cm* = middle turbinate; *be* = ethmoidal bulla; *pu* = uncinate process.

anterior extension of the bulla may completely obscure the middle turbinate, making the initial endoscopic diagnosis difficult.

More commonly there is a general enlargement of the ethmoidal bulla that completely fills the space under a somewhat laterally curled middle turbinate. In extreme cases this general enlargement of the bulla produces an extensive area of surface contact between the medial surface of bulla and the lateral mucosal surface of the middle turbinate (the "turbinate sinus"). In our experience, this is one of the most common sites from which nasal polyps originate.

An enlarged but otherwise nondiseased ethmoidal bulla can fill the entire middle meatus tightly, like a balloon, and give rise to significant symptoms. The most frequent symptoms produced in this situation are heavy and unpleasant pressure above or behind the eyes, impeded or blocked nasal breathing, or the feeling that something is stuck in the nose, causing a continuous sneezing or blowing urge without being able to blow anything out. A large or diseased ethmoidal bulla, by virtue of its areas of contact with the mucosal surfaces of adjacent structures, may also be responsible for a postnasal discharge. Headaches, especially frontal headaches, are frequently the chief complaint.

Because of its central location and its multiple intimate anatomic relationships to the other key areas of the anterior ethmoid, the ethmoidal bulla is frequently involved in those disease processes that affect the anterior ethmoid. Even minor mucosal swellings can affect the hiatus semilunaris and the ethmoidal infundibulum. The frontal recess, the agger nasi, and the lateral sinus all may become involved as well.

When assessing an ethmoidal bulla radiologically, one must remember that there need not be marked opacification of the bulla or of its immediate surroundings to identify the bulla as an etiologic factor in the disease process. A normally aerated but enlarged ethmoidal bulla may be the principal cause of the symptoms, as seen in Figure 4–16, where there are marked contact areas between the enlarged bulla and the middle turbinate. Through its extensive downward growth, this enlarged bulla has significantly narrowed the ethmoidal infundibulum and the ostium of the maxillary sinus. In this case, a radiographic report mentioning a "normally aerated ethmoid" is correct, but insufficient because it may lead to the conclusion that there is no pathologic process. This case emphasizes the importance of good communication between the otorhinolaryngologist and the radiologist.

LATERAL SINUS

The lateral sinus (sinus lateralis) is a highly variable space bounded by the ethmoidal bulla, the roof of the ethmoid, the basal lamella of the middle turbinate, and the lamina papyracea. Localized disease can develop within the lateral sinus without involving the ethmoidal bulla (Fig 4–18). Disease in the lateral sinus is usually difficult to diagnose endoscopically, and occasionally the only indication of a pathologic condition in this area is the observation of a small amount of abnormal secretions coming from the superior hiatus semilunaris. Small polyps or mucosal swellings that appear medial to the bulla and that exert pressure inferiorly may also indicate disease in the lateral sinus (Fig 4–19). If the lateral sinus is well developed and extends far posteriorly, the ethmoidal bulla may open into the lateral sinus, creating a pathway through which disease can spread from the bulla to the lateral sinus, and vice versa.

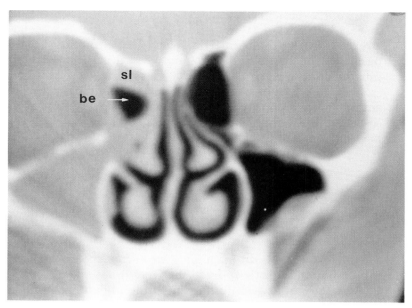

FIG 4–18.
Lateral sinus on the right is diseased. The turbinate sinus and the infundibulum are also involved, and disease has spread to the maxillary sinus. The ethmoidal bulla is only slightly involved. *si* = sinus lateralis; *be* = ethmoidal bulla.

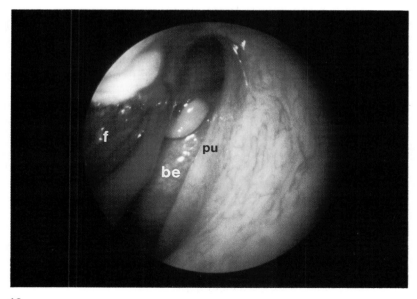

FIG 4–19.
In this patient the polyps originated from the superior hiatus semilunaris. They were a manifestation of involvement of the left lateral sinus. The slight pressure of the Freer elevator displacing the middle meatus medially has caused a small hemorrhage. *pu* = uncinate process; *be* = bulla ethmoidalis; *p* = polyp; *f* = Freer elevator.

In our experience, the lateral sinus is the ethmoidal fissure from which disease spreads most frequently across the basal lamella to the posterior ethmoid. This spread of infection occurs either through bony dehiscences of the basal lamella or through circumscribed areas of destruction as a result of inflammation.

Depending on its anatomic shape and relations, disease within the lateral sinus may spread to the frontal recess and to the agger nasi, and vice versa. The so-called supraorbital ethmoidal cells are usually only lateral extensions of the lateral sinus that extend deeply into the roof of the orbits.

DISEASES OF ETHMOIDAL INFUNDIBULUM

The majority of the drainage pathways from the anterior ethmoid join in the infundibulum with those from the frontal and maxillary sinuses, and consequently, the ethmoidal infundibulum (infundibulum ethmoidale) is the key area in inflammatory diseases of the paranasal sinuses. Because of its anatomic shape (long, narrow fissure), the patency of the infundibulum is affected early and rapidly by even minor and localized changes in the adjacent structures. Conversely, disease that develops primarily in the infundibulum can spread quickly to involve the adjacent structures, especially the larger frontal and maxillary sinuses.

Because the endoscopist's normal view is limited to the hiatus semilunaris and includes the infundibulum only in the rarest of instances, endoscopic diagnosis is limited to the recognition and evaluation of those physical signs that point directly or indirectly to the presence of infundibular disease.

A routine plain survey film of the sinuses for all practical purposes fails to show the area of the ethmoidal infundibulum, and thus the information provided by plain radiographs does not allow any conclusions to be drawn about the presence or absence of diseases in the infundibulum. This is the major reason we must combine diagnostic endoscopy with conventional tomography or CT to properly investigate sinus disease.

The diagnostic endoscopic examination provide the indications for tomography by the observation of direct or indirect evidence of infundibular disease, whereas tomograms will reveal those hidden disease processes that are not endoscopically visible. Tomograms also enable us to decide whether a more invasive diagnostic procedure or an endoscopic surgical procedure is indicated.

Four prime endoscopic clues suggest the presence of disease within the infundibulum:

1. Obvious pathologic changes in the infundibulum or the hiatus semilunaris.
2. Observation of pathologic secretions draining from the infundibulum via the hiatus semilunaris.
3. Identification of anatomic variants that are capable of constricting the infundibulum.
4. Observation of mucosal changes on the medial surface of the uncinate process that suggest infundibular disease.

The endoscopic or radiologic findings may uncover hidden disease in the infundibulum (Fig 4–20). Conversely, an impressive endoscopic finding need not necessarily be responsible for significant symptoms, as is frequently seen in patients who have a moderate number of nasal polyps. Although these patients may in some cases complain of partially obstructed nasal breathing, a limitation in the sense of smell, or of blockage of the eustachian tube, they frequently have no other serious symptoms.

All of these factors must be taken into account when a surgical procedure is being considered. Surgical procedures should never be undertaken on the basis of the radiologic findings alone, but should always be planned from careful assessment of the radiologic and endoscopic findings in combination with the clinical symptoms.

The endoscopic picture of infundibular disease is extremely variable because there is a continuous spectrum, from minor, isolated, and circumscribed disease to massive involvement of the entire ethmoid and related paranasal sinuses.

In relatively circumscribed disease the typical mucosal changes are best seen in the area of the hiatus semilunaris, where abnormal or adherent discharge provides evidence of disease within the infundibulum. If the disease spreads further within the infundibulum, one usually sees edematous, inflammatory changes in the mucosa of the free posterior margin of the uncinate process and on the anterior surface of the ethmoidal bulla. There may also be polypoid changes in both of these areas. Individual polyps or irregular mucosal folds may obstruct the infundibulum and the hiatus semilunaris and extend into the middle meatus to prolapse anteriorly or inferiorly. Depending on the nature of the disease process, the medial wall of the infundibulum (whose bony base consists of the uncinate process) may be displaced medially or anteriorly. This is often seen clearly in acute sinus infection.

The mucous membrane covering the medial surface of the uncinate process need not show any changes. At times, increased vascular markings are the only indication for an inflammatory process deep in the infundibulum.

Finally, an inflammatory edematous engorgement of the mucous membrane may be superimposed on an anterior bulging uncinate process. This is most commonly seen in chronic cases where the swollen mucosa frequently blocks the entrance to the middle meatus either partially or completely.

Granulomatous changes and polyps may also be seen, not only at the sites of contact between the wall of the uncinate process and the middle turbinate but also projecting anteriorly and inferiorly from the anterior surface of the ethmoidal bulla and from the more superior ethmoid fissures. The bony base of the uncinate process may be partially destroyed, and perforations may appear through the uncinate process into the middle meatus. Granulation tissue, polyps, or pathologic secretions may be seen emerging from these perforations. Figure 4–20 shows the typical endoscopic and radiologic findings of infundibular disease.

The symptoms of isolated infundibular disease are usually mild and nonspecific. Headaches, often only a mild, dull pressure between the eyes or in the area of the inner canthus, a feeling of fullness in the nose, and a sensation of impeded nasal breathing despite an open nasal passage, all are suggestive of infundibular disease. If the larger paranasal sinuses become secondarily involved by disease in the ethmoidal infundibulum, the clinical picture will be dominated by the symptoms originating in these larger sinuses.

A

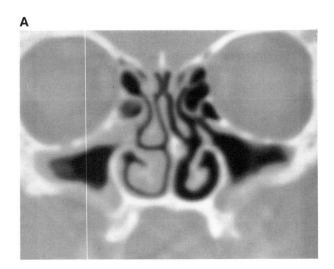

B

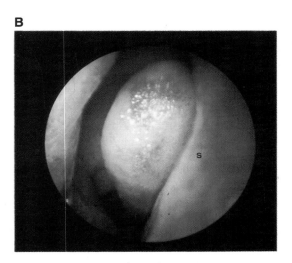

C

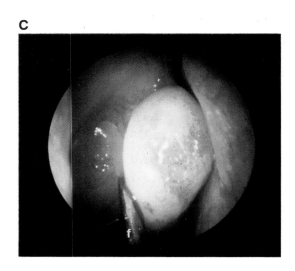

D

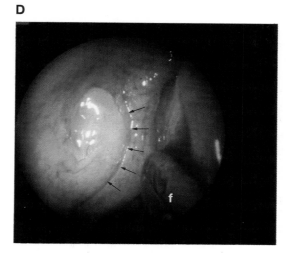

FIG 4–20.
A, typical CT of infundibular disease. (Clinically the chief complaint was recurrent maxillary sinusitis.) The infundibulum is blocked by edematous mucous membrane between the uncinate process, the bulla, and the lamina papyracea. Note the ensuing mucosal edema in the right maxillary sinus. **B,** at endoscopy, the swollen head of the middle turbinate obstructs the view into the middle meatus. **C,** after the turbinate has been carefully retracted medially, polypoid mucosa appears on the medial wall of the infundibulum where it and the turbinate were in contact. **D,** posterior edge of the uncinate process is in close contact with the bulla ethmoidalis and thus completely closes the hiatus semilunaris (*arrows*). *f* = Freer elevator.

DISEASES OF FRONTAL RECESS

The frontal recess is most commonly affected by disease that originates in the adjacent areas of the ostiomeatal complex, for example, in the ethmoidal infundibulum, hiatus semilunaris, sinus of the turbinate, or lateral sinus. Disease, however, can develop in the frontal recess as an isolated process. The involvement of the various compartments of the ethmoid by the internal spread of disease in the ethmoid depends not only on the type and virulence of the inflammatory process but also, most important, on the anatomic configuration of the individual components of the ethmoid.

Because the frontal recess is the ethmoidal prechamber of the frontal sinus, many of the changes that ultimately produce actual disease in the frontal sinus will be found in the frontal recess. Just as in the maxillary sinus, the frontal sinus is usually involved only secondarily, with infection reaching it through the nose by way of its prechamber (the frontal recess). Even when the symptoms of frontal sinusitis dominate the clinical picture, the source of these symptoms will usually be found not in the frontal sinus itself but in the adjacent ethmoidal sinus. It should be emphasized that when plain survey radiographs of the paranasal sinuses show opacities or an air fluid level in the frontal sinus, these changes are usually the result of a disease process in the frontal recess. Even when the frontal sinuses are extensively involved, the changes in the frontal recess may appear very slight and identified only by conventional tomography or CT.

The endoscopic findings may also be minimal in disease of the frontal sinus. Abnormal secretions arising from the middle meatus may be the only endoscopic indication of frontal recess disease. Depending on the shape of the uncinate process, these secretions may be carried directly to the infundibulum and appear only at the posterior portion of the hiatus semilunaris. From there they drain medially, across the uncinate process. Frequently, circumscribed inflammatory mucous membrane changes in the frontal recess can be detected only if a 30- or 70-degree nasal endoscope can be introduced into the middle meatus. Occasionally, small polyps may be seen extending forward and downward, just below the attachment of the middle turbinate. Larger polyps may bulge out of the middle meatus and block any view of the middle meatus or of the attachment of the middle turbinate. Inflammatory bulging of the uppermost portion of the uncinate process, spreading eventually to the mucosa over the attachment of the middle turbinate, may also be an indication of a disease process in the frontal recess, with incipient spread to the ethmoidal infundibulum.

If the drainage of secretions from the frontal recess (and thus from the frontal sinus) is completely blocked, a mucocele or a pyocele may develop from the retained secretions. In such cases the medial wall of the frontal recess (i.e., that part of the middle turbinate immediately above the most anterior part of its attachment) may be bulging medially and may even come into contact with the nasal septum. The mucous membrane in this area may be only minimally affected, although increased vascular markings frequently will be observed over the protruding area. Inflammatory changes and polyp formation at the point of contact with the septum are not rare. Mucosal engorgement and polyp formation in this area are a common cause of obstruction of the olfactory fissure. In the case of a frontal sinus empyema, it may be possible to initiate the drainage of the pathologic secretions by placing a decongestant pledget directly into the frontal recess.

Diseases of the frontal recess do not necessarily produce all of the symptoms of a frontal sinus infection, and frequently the prime complaints are limited to an unpleasant sensation of pressure in the inner canthus or over the inferomedial aspect of the frontal sinus, and most commonly frontal headache. In such patients it is important to perform a careful endoscopic examination of the frontal recess when the examiner suspects that the symptoms are the result of frontal recess disease. This is particularly important when the plain films are normal. Because it may be impossible to inspect the frontal recess, even with the slender 2.7-mm diameter endoscope, the examiner should attempt to view the frontal recess by displacing the middle turbinate medially with a Freer elevator or by using the Messerklinger technique of introducing the endoscope through a small trocar sheath.

Almost all of the anatomic variations of the structures of the anterior ethmoid can produce stenosis in the area of the frontal recess. Prominent among these variations are those of the uncinate process, the ethmoidal bulla, the formation of a concha bullosa of the middle turbinate, or marked pneumatization of the agger nasi cells. Fig 4–21 demonstrates a variety of endoscopic and radiographic findings in frontal recess disease.

Endoscopic diagnosis has proved valuable in the conservative medical therapy of primary, acute frontal sinusitis. In these patients the examiner can usually pinpoint the etiologic focus of disease in the frontal recess. In patients with frontal sinus empyema or with an air fluid level, one can usually introduce a topical decongestant, with or without the addition of a topical anesthetic, right into the frontal recess, under direct endoscopic control. This usually results in improvement of the symptoms by promoting drainage of secretions. When it is combined with simultaneous antibiotic therapy, most cases of acute frontal sinusitis can be managed conservatively. If these maneuvers do not produce

A

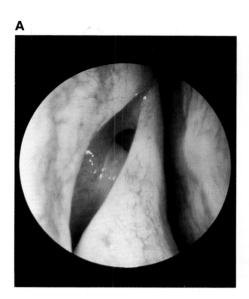

B

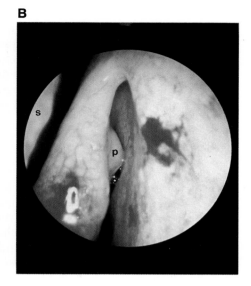

C

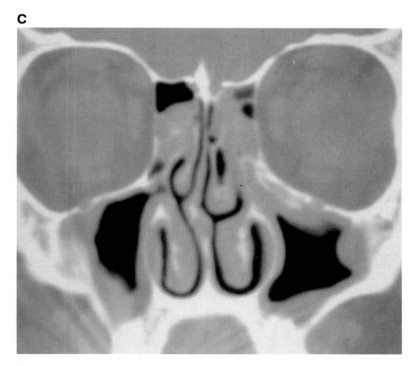

FIG 4–21.
A, this apparently small polyp emerging from the frontal recess directly below the insertion of the right middle turbinate was visible only on endoscopic examination. **B,** on the left side of the patient, there was a similar, presumably minor finding. *s* = septum; *p* = polyps. **C,** because this patient had therapy resistant complaints for many years (primarily headaches and recurrent frontal and maxillary sinusitis), tomography was performed. The tomograms revealed significant disease of the ethmoidal infundibulum bilaterally, with spread to the frontal recess.

definite improvement in the symptoms or if the symptoms recur promptly after a period of improvement, we perform tomography, and if indicated, an endoscopic surgical exploration of the frontal recess. Only in rare cases (e.g., threat of complications such as incipient osteomyelitis or intracranial complications) do we resort to an external surgical approach. Since we started using this conservative endoscopic technique during the past decade, we have not had to perform trephination of the frontal sinus.

AGGER NASI

A pneumatized agger nasi is an anatomic variant that appears as an elevation of the lateral wall of the nose just anterior to the attachment of the middle turbinate. Endoscopically the agger nasi can appear as a small eminence just anterior to the insertion of the middle turbinate. In some persons the agger does not rise above the surrounding structures. The agger nasi is considered an anatomic variant when it becomes pneumatized, usually from the frontal recess, to form the agger nasi cells. When there is extensive pneumatization, an enlarged agger nasi air cell may displace the attachment of the middle turbinate medially and superiorly. When this occurs, the agger may appear as a distinct bulge on endoscopy (Fig 4–22). When an agger nasi cell is very large or if it extends posteriorly, it may mechanically constrict the frontal recess.

From a clinical diagnostic perspective, it is important to remember that the agger nasi cells abut laterally onto the paper thin lacrimal bone, which can have dehiscences. Any disease process within the agger nasi can therefore easily extend to the adjacent lacrimal sac, causing epiphora or other inflammatory conditions of the lacrimal system. When the ophthalmologist is unable to find local causes for such conditions, an endoscopic examination, and if indicated,

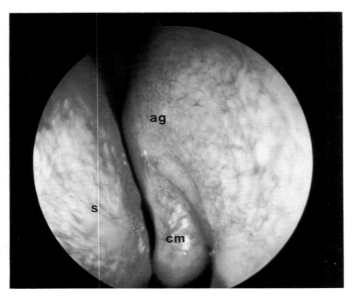

FIG 4–22.
An agger nasi cell can be seen arching the lateral nasal wall above and anterior to the insertion of the middle turbinate. The uncinate process is slightly bent medially. *s* = septum; *cm* = middle turbinate; *ag* = agger nasi area.

tomography, may reveal the underlying intranasal cause. The symptoms arising from isolated agger nasi cell disease may be atypical, and usually there is only a sensation of pressure between the eyes, with tenderness or pain over the medial palpebral ligament.

Involvement of the agger nasi cells by disease processes of the frontal recess or of the ethmoidal infundibulum occurs more commonly than isolated agger nasi pathologic conditions. Depending on the anatomic configuration, there may be a connection between the agger nasi and the lateral sinus, and consequently disease may spread between these two areas. Large but otherwise healthy agger nasi cells may by themselves be a frequent cause of disease in the frontal recess. We have repeatedly found enlarged agger nasi cells as the sole etiologic factor in divers and aviators who have experienced difficulty in equalizing pressure changes.

Endoscopically, marked bulging of the lateral nasal wall anterior and sometimes superior to the attachment of the middle turbinate may indicate disease in the agger nasi. These endoscopic findings are significant only when the changes are pronounced. Definitive diagnosis of disease in the agger nasi can be made only with tomograms taken in the coronal plane (Fig 4–23). Coronal views clearly demonstrate the anatomic relationship of the agger nasi to the lacrimal fossa. In coronal sections, those cells seen below the level of the frontal sinus and frontal recess and that are located anterior to the attachment of the middle turbinate are the agger nasi cells.

If the agger nasi is opacified, delineation of their posterior limit may be difficult, because in some patients the agger nasi may have a wide communication with the frontal recess and even with the lateral sinus. If the distance between sections is greater than 4 mm, the next section may cut through the ethmoidal bulla beyond the agger, making the radiologic separation between these two structures difficult.

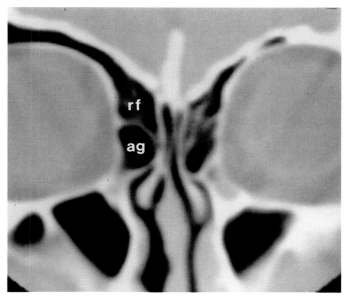

FIG 4–23.
In this tomogram, bilateral large agger nasi cells are seen constricting (by their size) the frontal recess from inferiorly. *rf* = frontal recess; *ag* = agger nasi.

HALLER CELLS

Haller cells are another anatomic variant that may play an important role in the development of maxillary sinusitis. Haller cells are ethmoidal cells that develop into the floor of the orbit (i.e., the roof of the maxillary sinus) adjacent to and above the natural ostium of the maxillary sinus. When enlarged, Haller cells can significantly constrict the posterior aspect of the ethmoidal infundibulum and the ostium of the maxillary sinus from above. If a Haller cell becomes diseased, the natural ostium of the maxillary sinus may rapidly become obstructed and secondary maxillary sinusitis develop.

Changes secondary to infundibular disease, such as slight bulging in the lateral nasal wall below the ethmoidal bulla and narrowing of the most posterior part of the hiatus semilunaris, may suggest the presence of a Haller cell. However, because Haller cells are located lateral to the infundibulum, they cannot be identified by nasal diagnostic endoscopy. During endoscopic examination of the maxillary sinus (sinuscopy), on the other hand, the presence of an enlarged or diseased Haller cell is usually obvious (Fig 4–24).

The diagnosis of a Haller cell is thus made primarily by tomography. Figure 4–25 clearly shows the presence of a large pneumatized Haller cell constricting the ostium of the maxillary sinus. This radiograph shows how even minor swelling of the mucous membranes (from any cause) can block the ostium of the maxillary sinus completely.

DISEASES OF POSTERIOR ETHMOIDAL SINUS

The posterior ethmoidal sinus is located, by definition, in the area bounded by the basal lamella of the middle turbinate anteroinferiorly, the lamina papyracea of the orbit laterally, and the superior or supreme turbinate medially. Posteriorly the posterior ethmoidal sinus may extend not only up to the anterior wall of the sphenoidal sinus but, in some individuals, may extend by means of a special cellular projection (Onodi cells) laterally well beyond the sphenoid sinus (see Fig 2–5).

Isolated inflammatory diseases of the posterior ethmoidal sinus are extremely rare. In our patients, disease in the posterior ethmoidal sinuses is usually combined with disease in the anterior ethmoidal sinus, and less commonly with disease of the sphenoidal sinus. The posterior ethmoidal sinus is most frequently involved in diffuse polypoid sinusitis. Otherwise the posterior ethmoidal sinus is involved in only about one third of those cases of chronic sinusitis of inflammatory origin (see Table 4–1).

Endoscopically, a drainage of secretions from the superior or supreme meatus or from the sphenoethmoidal recess may be the only indication of posterior ethmoidal sinus disease (Fig 4–26). Inflamed or polypoid mucosa may protrude from the superior or supreme meatus.

In our experience, those larger polyps, which appear between the middle turbinate and the nasal septum, may have three sites of origin: the mucosa of the olfactory fissure in cases of diffuse polyposis; the site of mucosal contact between the nasal septum and the middle turbinate, or less commonly with the superior turbinate (arising from either the septum or the turbinate); or from the posterior ethmoidal sinus, with the polyps extending anteriorly and medially through the superior meatus to appear in the nasal cavity medial to the middle turbinate. In severe polyposis, polyps originating from the posterior ethmoidal

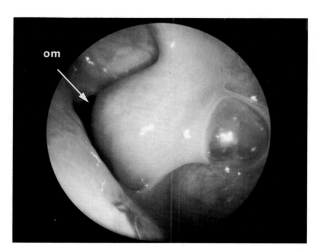

FIG 4–24.
This is the endoscopic finding inside a left maxillary sinus. The bulging of the Haller cell from the roof of the orbit can be clearly seen. The ostium of the maxillary sinus is severely constricted by this large cell (*arrow*). After the empyema is removed by suction, residual foamy secretions can still be seen along the Haller cell. *om* = maxillary sinus ostium.

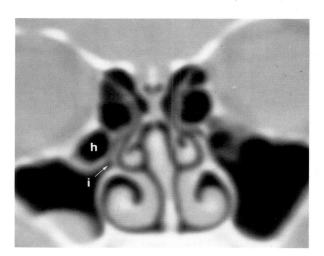

FIG 4–25.
Tomogram showing bilateral Haller's cells with obvious narrowing of the ethmoidal infundibulum on the right side (*arrow*). *i* = infundibulum; *h* = Haller's cell.

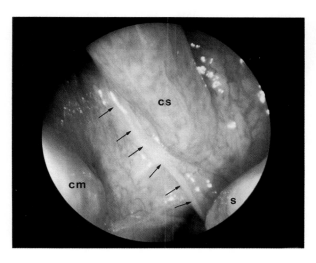

FIG 4–26.
Tenacious secretions in the right superior meatus (*arrows*) suggest posterior ethmoidal sinus disease. *cm* = posterior end of the middle turbinate; *cs* = superior turbinate; *s* = posterior end of the septum.

sinus and from the margin of the superior turbinate are frequently found in the sphenoethmoidal recess.

If the posterior ethmoidal sinus is extensively pneumatized, and especially if the pneumatization extends laterally along the sphenoidal sinus, the posterolateral portions of the posterior ethmoidal sinus may come into intimate contact with the optic nerve (see Fig 2–5). We have encountered cases where the optic nerve, covered only by a very thin layer of bone, passed almost freely through the posterior ethmoidal sinus (i.e., the optic nerve was surrounded by pneumatic spaces both medially and laterally). This possibility must always be kept in mind during surgery for diffuse nasal polyposis. These Onodi cells cannot always be identified accurately by endoscopy, and only tomography can identify these cells and their relationship to the optic nerve with certainty. Changing the plane of the tomographic examination can clearly show the ocular muscles, the course of the optic nerve, and its relationship to the posterior ethmoidal sinus, particularly on axial CT scans.

In extensive pneumatization, both the sphenoidal sinus and the posterior ethmoidal sinus may be in close contact with the foramen rotundum. In rare cases, the foramen rotundum may even be surrounded by pneumatized spaces laterally. In this situation, the second division of the trigeminal nerve can become involved when the posterior portion of the posterior ethmoidal sinus becomes diseased.

Because even the root of the pterygoid process may be reached by extensive pneumatization, this area and the critical structures it contains may also become involved in inflammatory diseases of the posterior ethmoidal sinus. The same is also true for the nerve of the pterygoid canal (vidian nerve). In midface neuralgias, the possibility of an irritation of the second division of the trigeminal nerve, originating from the posterior ethmoidal sinus, should be considered. Figure 4–27 shows the typical radiographic findings in disease of the posterior ethmoidal sinus.

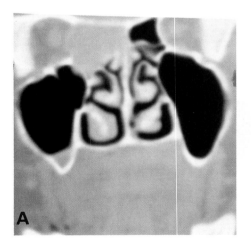 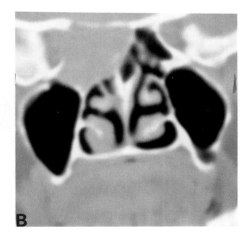

FIG 4–27.
A, and **B,** in this CT scan, the homogeneous opacification of the right posterior ethmoid is a large mucocele that includes the posterior ethmoid and the maxillary sinus. The medial wall of the orbital apex has been destroyed. The mucocele caused blindness and ophthalmoplegia in this patient. The ophthalmoplegia disappeared postoperatively, but, unfortunately, the vision could not be restored.

DISEASES OF SPHENOIDAL SINUS

The sphenoidal sinus is involved in only about 16% of patients with chronic sinusitis. Most of the time these are not separate diseases but contiguous involvement from disease in the adjacent posterior ethmoidal sinus, which produces secondary edema of the mucous membranes of the sphenoidal sinus that appears as opacification on tomograms. Isolated involvement of the sphenoidal sinus is nevertheless more frequent than that of the posterior ethmoidal sinus. These involvements may include mucoceles, pyoceles, or isolated fungal infections.

Clinically the most prominent symptom is headache, which is usually central, occasionally radiating to the temples or to the crown of the head. The most common endoscopic findings are the presence of a variable amount of secretion discharged through the sphenoidal recess into the nasopharynx (Figs 4–28 and 4–29).

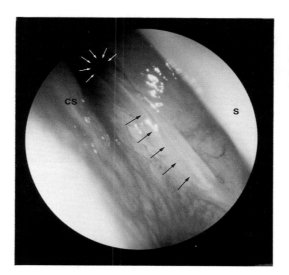

FIG 4–28.
Note the viscous, mucopurulent secretions (*black arrows*) draining into the sphenoethmoidal recess from the ostium of a right sphenoidal sinus (*white arrows*). *cs* = superior turbinate; *s* = septum.

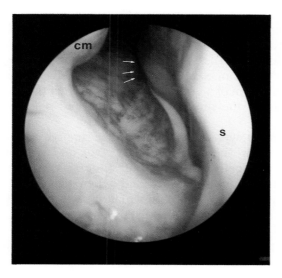

FIG 4–29.
In this patient, purulent secretions can be seen draining from the right sphenoidal sinus through the sphenoethmoidal recess and on to the choana. After the insertion of decongestant pledgets, the sphenoidal ostium (*arrows*) can be seen as a narrow fissure. The superior turbinate cannot be seen. *s* = septum; *cm* = dorsal end of the middle turbinate.

In most cases the examiner can without too much difficulty obtain an endoscopic view into the sphenoethmoidal recess by using a 2.7-mm 30- or 70-degree endoscope. Even when it is not possible to look directly at the ostium of the sphenoidal sinus, changes can usually be identified that suggest the presence of sphenoidal sinus disease. The observation of highly viscous or even frankly purulent secretions or mucosal swellings of variable severity, which may even completely obstruct the sphenoethmoidal recess, are all important clinical findings that suggest the presence of sphenoidal sinus disease.

Once the type and extent of the sphenoidal sinus disease have been radiologically established, the other major points of interest on the tomograms are the relationship of the sphenoidal sinus to the optic nerve and to the bulge of the internal carotid artery. During surgical procedures on the sphenoidal sinus, the surgeon must always remember that both the optic canal and the bulge of the internal carotid artery may be covered by only a very thin and occasionally fragmented bony layer in the area of the sphenoidal sinus and that these two vital structures may not be well protected. In addition, the surgeon must always be aware that the internal carotid artery may bulge far into the lumen of the sphenoidal sinus.

Depending on the degree of pneumatization, both the foramen rotundum and the pterygoid canal may protrude into the lumen of the sphenoidal sinus. If the bony walls of the sphenoidal sinus have been damaged, these nerves can become affected by the disease process in the sinus. It is therefore important to remember the possible etiologic relationship between a disease process in the ethmoidal or sphenoidal sinuses and the wide variety of facial pains or "atypical trigeminal neuralgia" that could be cured by endoscopic means once the proper diagnosis is made.

Isolated polyps originating from the anterior wall of the sphenoidal sinus or from its interior and extending as choanal polyps into the nasopharynx are extremely rare.

NASAL POLYPOSIS

Nasal polyposis is the most common chronic disease affecting the mucous membranes of the nasal cavity and the paranasal sinuses, and following chronic sinusitis, nasal polyposis is the most frequent indication for surgical intervention in the nose and paranasal sinuses.

The cause of polyp formation is still widely debated. Only one common denominator, mucosal edema, can be proved in the cause of nasal polyps. Even today there is no clear definition of a "nasal polyp," and in fact the dividing line between localized edema of the mucous membranes and a polyp remains unclear.

When we speak of nasal polyposis, we must realize that we are not dealing with a single disease entity; there are at least two, and probably more, clinically and pathophysiologically distinct manifestations. This must be taken into consideration when planning therapy and when evaluating different treatment methods. Until we have better information, we must differentiate "normal," primarily inflammatory nasal polyposis from "diffuse, polypoid rhinosinopathy."

Clinically, nasal polyposis encompasses a wide spectrum, from circumscribed mucosal edema, through isolated polyps, to diffuse and massive polyposis that completely fills the nasal cavity and the paranasal sinuses. There is frequently a marked discrepancy between the symptoms and the clinical findings, and it is surprising how frequently patients with extensive nasal polyposis report relatively few symptoms, whereas other patients with relatively circumscribed, polypoid changes may have significant symptoms. The clinical appearance of nasal polyps may vary widely, from edematous to glassy, to cystic, coarse, and fibrotic.

Endoscopically it has been shown with few exceptions that almost all polyps that appear in the nasal cavity arise from the ethmoidal sinus or from its immediate vicinity. In uncomplicated nasal polyposis, the anterior ethmoidal sinus is almost always involved. With the exception of isolated choanal polyps or adjacent to tumors, we have not seen an isolated polyp arising from the posterior ethmoidal sinus.

Those patients in whom no gross polyps can be seen in the nasal cavity create special diagnostic demands on the endoscopist. The small polyp, illustrated in Figure 4–21, that protruded between the uncinate process and the attachment of the middle turbinate could not be seen with either the naked eye or a microscope and was detected with the endoscope only after the instrument was introduced into the nose as close as possible to the entrance to the middle meatus. At the time of this endoscopic examination, no additional abnormalities were seen in the nasal cavity. The plain sinus radiographs showed "normal" maxillary, frontal, and ethmoidal sinuses. In view of the long history of symptoms and the presumably minor endoscopic findings, tomography was performed, which showed opacities in the infundibulum and in the frontal recess. At surgery, surprisingly large polypoid masses were removed from this area of the ethmoidal sinus, where they had apparently exerted considerable pressure, thereby contributing significantly to the patient's symptoms. In this case, the tiny polyp discovered during the endoscopic examination represented only the tip of the iceberg.

Even in severe polyposis, the site of origin of the polyps in the middle meatus can frequently be identified. Table 4–1 displays the findings that we have gathered in 200 patients during endoscopic examination or surgery. It is evident that the majority of the polyps originated in the narrow spaces of the

TABLE 4–1

Origination of Polyps in 200 Consecutive Patients*

Primary sinuses affected
80%   Uncinate—turbinate—infundibulum
65%   Face of bulla—hiatus—infundibulum
48%   Frontal recess
42%   "Turbinate sinus"
30%   Inside bulla
28%   "Lateral sinus"
27%   Posterior ethmoidal sinus (superior meatus)
15%   Middle turbinate
Secondary sinuses affected
65%   Maxillary sinus (mucosal swelling)
23%   Frontal sinus (mucosal swelling)
 8%   Sphenoid sinus

* Does not include diffuse polypoid rhinosinopathy.

(anterior) ethmoidal sinus (Fig 4–30). The most frequent sites of origin were the contact areas of the uncinate process and the middle turbinate and the ethmoidal infundibulum. Eighty percent of our patients had polyps originating from these areas.

In almost two thirds of patients, polyps also originated from the anterior aspect of the ethmoidal bulla, where they obstructed the hiatus semilunaris, invaded the ethmoidal infundibulum, or protruded anteriorly between the middle turbinate and the uncinate process into the middle meatus.

In about 50% of the patients, polyps were discovered in the frontal recess. This is particularly important, because often in this area the polyps may not be visible even through the endoscope. It is in this situation that the combination of diagnostic endoscopy and tomography is especially valuable.

A

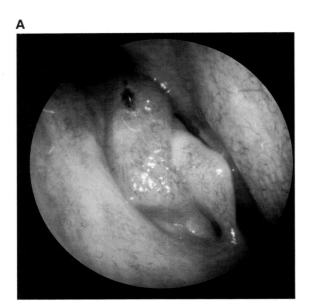

FIG 4–30.
A, a large polyp can be seen extruding from the left middle meatus. **B,** when the polyp is displaced medially by a Freer elevator, the origin of the polyp can be seen. It arises by a stalk from the anterior and inferior surface of the ethmoidal bulla, as well as from the topmost portion of the uncinate process.

B

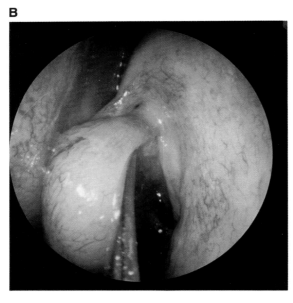

Other common sites of origin were the turbinate sinus (the space between the concavity of the middle turbinate and the medial surface of the ethmoidal bulla (42% of all patients) and the lateral sinus (the variably developed space between the roof of the ethmoid superiorly, the ethmoidal bulla inferiorly, the basal lamella of the middle turbinate posteriorly, the lamina papyracea laterally, and the middle turbinate medially). The lateral sinus was most frequently affected when there was a simultaneous polypoid involvement of the posterior ethmoid.

Sixty-five percent of patients had a variable degree of mucous membrane engorgement in the maxillary sinus, and 23% in the frontal sinus. Except for a few patients with retention cysts, we found no significant maxillary or frontal sinus disease in which there was not also a pathologic process in the adjacent areas of the ethmoid. Polypoid changes in the sphenoidal sinus were found in only 8% of patients.

It is apparent that polyps originate much more frequently from the fissures and narrow spaces of the ethmoid than from the ethmoidal cells themselves. Such precise identification of the site of origin is not possible if the polyposis is massive or is recurrent after surgical extirpation.

Those polyps visible *medial to the middle turbinate* (Fig 4–31) usually originate from one of three sites:

1. Mucous membrane of the olfactory fissure (extremely rare except in cases of diffuse polypoid rhinosinopathy).
2. Contact area between the middle turbinate and the nasal septum.
3. Posterior ethmoid or from the superior meatus, from where they prolapse and thus lie medial to the middle turbinate.

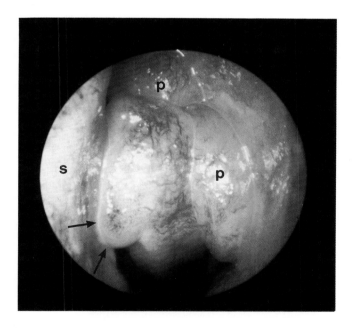

FIG 4–31.
In this patient there is a large concha bullosa of the left middle turbinate, and polyps can be seen extruding from the middle meatus. There are also polypoid mucous membrane changes (*arrows*) at the area of contact between the concha bullosa and the nasal septum. *p* = polyps; *s* = septum.

Polyps may prolapse into the sphenoethmoidal recess from the posterior ethmoidal sinus in a similar manner. Isolated polyps arising from the sphenoidal sinus are extremely rare.

In those patients with massive polyposis it may not be possible to advance the endoscope to the entrance of the middle meatus, especially when the polyps have extended into the vestibule of the nose. In even more severe polyposis, there may be a polypoid, lobular hyperplasia of the head or of the free margin of the middle turbinate. We have encountered this type of polypoidal degeneration in about 15% of our patients with severe polyposis.

The degree of mucosal disease in the maxillary or frontal sinuses does not correlate with the total *mass* of ethmoidal polyps. Total opacification from retained secretions of these larger paranasal sinuses can occur in the presence of only circumscribed ethmoidal disease.

We have found that it is not the extent of the ethmoidal polyps that determines the involvement of the maxillary and frontal sinuses but the location of these changes. When the maxillary and frontal sinuses were opacified, we were almost always able to demonstrate secondary disease in the adjacent connected key sites of the lateral wall of the nose.

When considering the indications for surgical intervention, the surgeon must remember that a significant percentage of the radiographic shadows in the maxillary sinus are simply due to retained secretions. These retained secretions are extremely viscous and have a curved radiographic contour that frequently cannot be distinguished from cystic or polypoid changes. Assessment of the interior of the maxillary sinus may be possible only at surgery, either through an enlarged ostium in the middle meatus or by perioperative endoscopy through the canine fossa. Not infrequently cysts and polyps extend from the ethmoid, through the ostium and into the maxillary sinus. In view of these facts, there is usually little need for direct surgical intervention directed primarily toward the frontal and maxillary sinuses.

In patients with sinubronchial syndrome (bronchial asthma and chronic sinusitis), especially of the aspirin-sensitive variety, extremely viscous secretions are usually found between the polyps. Because of its high viscosity and surface tension, these secretions frequently assume a globular shape and cannot always be distinguished from polyps, even by endoscopy (Fig 4–32). In some

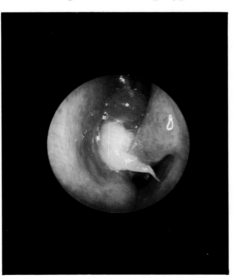

FIG 4–32.
Large, white polypoid mass seen adjacent to the inferior turbinate in the left nasal cavity is in fact abnormally thick, tenacious mucoid secretion. Note the polyp above the mucus, which originated in the middle meatus. This figure shows the classic appearance of the ASA triad.

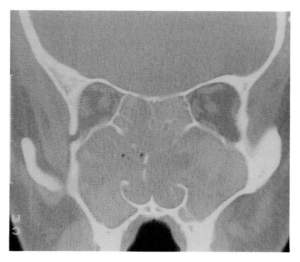

FIG 4–33.
Total opacification of the paranasal sinuses seen in this posterior coronal CT scan shows the classic "white-out" appearance of the ASA triad. In this patient the opacifications in the maxillary sinus and posterior ethmoid consisted of thick collections of inspissated mucus, and not polyps.

instances the mucus thread can be pulled out by the aspirator for a distance of 10 cm without breaking. Such tenacious mucus is found frequently in diseased sinuses, particularly in patients with asthma. Occasionally it is only during extraction that one notices that the forceps have grasped a mucous plug rather than a polyp. The production of this highly viscous secretion is a manifestation of a mucous membrane disorder of unknown cause.

CT scans are frequently difficult to interpret accurately in patients with recurrent nasal polyposis who have undergone previous surgical procedures and in those patients with nasal polyps who have a significant degree of retention of highly viscous secretions. The chronic inflammatory stimuli and possibly the pressure from the polyps may have caused extensive destruction of the thin bony septa and cellular walls of the ethmoidal region. Because of the slight differences in radiopacity, the entire nose and sinuses may appear to be homogeneously opacified all the way to the sphenoid sinus. Although this diffuse opacification suggests the need for a radical operation, in fact the cause of these opacities may be only moderate polyposis with corresponding stasis and retention that can be managed with a considerably less radical surgery. The indications for surgical intervention in general and for a radical procedure in particular should never be determined exclusively on the basis of radiologic findings (Fig 4–33).

Endoscopic Surgery for Polypoid Rhinosinusitis

Some nasal polyps can be cystic or extremely gelatinous. In this event, during their removal a clear watery liquid may seem to be mixed with the blood droplets in the surgical area. This makes the novice insecure, because it suggests a CSF leak. In contrast to the CSF leak, however, this type of clear liquid flow stops after a few seconds or at the latest when the corresponding polyp or cyst has been removed.

Difficulties may be encountered during surgery for recurrent nasal polyposis. In addition to the difficult anatomic conditions caused by the absence of the important topographic landmarks, the combination of polyps and scar tissue may be extremely coarse. If these are attached to the lamina papyracea or to the roof of the ethmoid, the greatest caution is required. Under no circumstances should these polyp-scar combinations be handled roughly in the vicinity of the base of the skull. Sometimes it is not possible to tell whether these scars are adherent to the dura. Two of the three CSF fistulas seen in our institution were in patients who had undergone several previous procedures for recurrent polyposis. We consider it entirely proper in such cases, for reasons of safety, to leave such fibrotic plaques alone, even with a few coarse polyps attached, and the patient must be informed accordingly.

Diffuse Polypoid Rhinosinopathy

One specific form of nasal polyposis, diffuse polypoid rhinosinopathy, has a distinct endoscopic appearance and clinical course, and must be distinguished from the types of nasal polyps previously described. Diffuse polypoid rhinosinopathy is a disease of unknown cause that represents generalized involvement of the entire nasal and paranasal sinus mucosa. In diffuse polypoid rhinosinopathy (Fig 4–34), the individual polyps can no longer be distinguished, and the diffusely engorged, polypoid mucous membrane of the middle meatus becomes confluent with the head and free margin of the middle turbinate and with the adjacent mucosal areas. The entire mucous membrane is so edematous and engorged that identification of individual landmarks is usually impossible. Tomography shows a homogeneous opacification of the entire nasal cavity or at least of the ethmoidal area. The frontal and maxillary sinuses are frequently

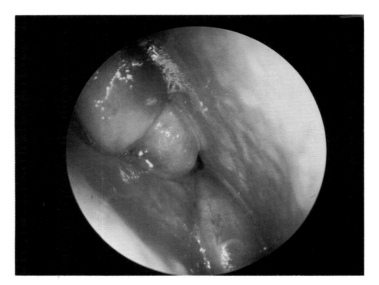

FIG 4–34.
Diffuse polypoid rhinosinopathy. Intranasal view in the direction of the olfactory fissure, on the right side, anterior to the insertion of the middle turbinate. The fissure is completely obstructed. This picture was taken after extensive local (topical) decongestion.

affected. Maxillary sinus endoscopy usually reveals diffuse swelling and polypoid degeneration of the entire mucous membranes (see Fig 4–34). These patients usually demonstrate no evidence of an IgE-mediated, type 1 allergy. Diffuse polypoid rhinosinopathy occurs more frequently in patients with aspirin sensitivity, asthma, or cystic fibrosis (see Fig 4–34).

Diffuse polypoid rhinosinopathy presents a major therapeutic problem because the diffuse changes in the mucous membranes are not particularly conducive to conservative medical therapy, yet when treated surgically, these patients have the highest recurrence rate, with symptoms frequently reappearing after only a few weeks (See Chapter 10). To date no effective medical therapy has been found, and even radical surgical procedures do not produce a permanent cure. In our experience, the largest percentage of therapeutic failures is in this group of patients.

Recurrent Nasal Polyps

A problem of particular concern to the surgeon is recurrent nasal polyps that develop after previous surgery. Depending on the type and number of previous operations, important landmarks such as the entire middle turbinate may be absent and the space between the lamina papyracea, the roof of the ethmoidal sinus, the cribriform plate, and the septum may be filled with dense fibrous adhesions surrounding a few polyps. In many cases even CT is unable to identify the structures so important that the surgeon be able to see.

During repeat surgical procedures the greatest caution is required, because the previous operation may have left significant bony defects at critical locations. Polyps on connective tissue strands may be attached to the dura of the cribriform plate or to the lamina papyracea. An attempt to remove these polyps may result in injury to these structures and the very real possibility of serious complications. Such preexisting bony defects may have resulted in prolapse of the orbital contents into the anterior or posterior ethmoidal sinus. Because of their approximately similar tissue density, such prolapsed orbital contents cannot be radiologically distinguished from diseased edematous mucous membranes. There is consequently a real risk of opening the orbit when attempting to remove what appears to be diseased mucous membrane from this area of the ethmoid.

Choanal Polyps

Although the cause of choanal polyps is unclear, they present a fairly uniform clinical picture. Antrochoanal polyps have two components. A cystic component frequently completely fills the maxillary sinus. This maxillary sinus component extends by a usually slender stalk through either the natural ostium of the maxillary sinus or, more commonly, through an accessory ostium in the posterior fontanelle to reach the middle meatus. There it becomes a solid polyp that, as it enlarges, fills the floor of the nose and reaches the choana. Depending on its size, the intranasal component of the polyp may reach the nasopharynx, where it may completely obstruct the choana and occasionally become visible through the mouth below the free margin of the soft palate.

This arrangement was found in more than 80% of choanal polyps in our surgical series. The point of origin in the maxillary sinus was almost always the posterior wall in the vicinity of the maxilloethmoidal angle. A second point of attachment was found in more than 50% of cases where the stalk of the polyp emerged from the maxillary sinus (i.e., at the posteroinferior part of the exit ostium). In about 70% of our patients the choanal polyp left the maxillary sinus through an accessory ostium in the posterior fontanelle; in only 29% did the natural ostium serve this purpose. Even in these latter cases, we could never be certain that the pressure exerted by the stalk of the polyp did not cause the preexisting accessory ostium to merge into the natural ostium.

Choanal polyps occur most frequently in children and young adults. They are usually unilateral, and can be diagnosed easily with a nasal endoscope. In polyps that extend into the nasopharynx, one can easily observe the mechanical stresses to which these polyps are subjected during deglutition and talking. On endoscopy, choanal polyps appear to have an hourglass shape, with the stalk riding on the inferior and posterior circumference of the accessory ostium (Figs 4–35 and 4–36).

A

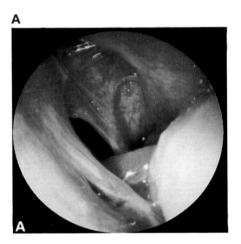

B

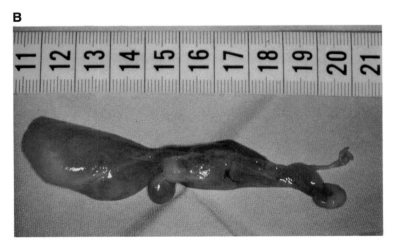

FIG 4–35.
A, the stalk of a choanal polyp that extends on the right side through a large accessory ostium in the posterior fontanelle to the nasopharynx. **B,** corresponding surgical specimen. On the right, the collapsed cystic component. On the left, the solid part of the polyp that had extended into the nasopharynx.

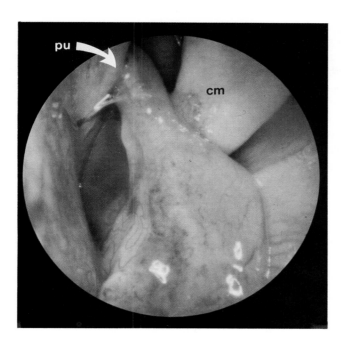

FIG 4–36.
This choanal polyp had only a small cystic component in the maxillary sinus and extended through the natural ostium, the infundibulum, and the hiatus semilunaris into the nasopharynx. The stalk appears from behind the uncinate process (*arrow*). *pu* = uncinate process; *cm* = middle turbinate.

Not all choanal polyps arise from the maxillary sinus; rarely, they may originate from the turbinate sinus, the anteroinferior surface of the ethmoidal bulla, the sphenoethmoidal recess, and, in one of our cases, the sphenoidal sinus. In none of these patients was the maxillary sinus involved.

A true antrochoanal polyp must be distinguished from polyps that extend to the choanae as part of a generalized nasal polyposis. One may occasionally see a combination of true choanal polyps and generalized polyposis of the ethmoidal sinuses.

Choanal polyps are a classic indication for endoscopic surgery, with very good prognosis and very low recurrence rate. However, choanal polyps have a high incidence of recurrence unless all of their components are carefully and completely removed. Recurrence is most common when mucosal remnants are allowed to remain at the site of origin in the maxillary sinus.

Endoscopic Surgery for Antrochoanal Polyps

The first step in the surgical procedure is endoscopic examination of the maxillary sinus through the fossa canina. Introduction of the maxillary sinus trocar usually breaks open the cystic portion of the polyps and allows suction removal of their contents. Any remaining cyst can be punctured with a sharpened polyethylene catheter and its wall removed through the trocar sheath. If the stalk of the polyp exits from the maxillary sinus through an accessory ostium in the posterior fontanelle, it may not be necessary to remove the uncinate process to resect the polyp.

DIFFERENTIAL DIAGNOSIS

A significant number of specific and nonspecific infections as well as benign and malignant neoplasms may involve the nose and paranasal sinuses. These diseases may produce typical and diagnostically pathognomonic changes as well as atypical nonspecific changes in the mucous membranes.

Messerklinger, in his classic text *Endoscopy of the Nose*, assembled a representative collection of endoscopic appearances and differential diagnoses of a large number of these diseases. A careful study of this outstanding work is recommended for all who engage in nasal endoscopy. At this time we wish to discuss the differential diagnostic aspects of nasal endoscopy that may be of value in differentiating malignant disease from chronic inflammation.

It is not always possible to identify specific diseases so clearly as the mucous membrane changes in sarcoidosis. Frequently the changes are so subtle that there appears to be no indication for biopsy before initiating medical therapy or even performing surgery. This was the case in Figure 4–37, where a relatively benign clinical appearance concealed a highly active tubercular lesion. It is particularly important in mycotic infections to remember that fungi can appear not only as harmless parasites on encrusted secretions but frequently on the ulcerated surfaces of malignant growths. For this reason the mucous membrane under a mycotic growth must be examined carefully and a biopsy performed.

Once there is tissue destruction and diffuse invasion, malignant processes usually have a characteristic radiographic appearance. It should be remembered, however, that chronic inflammatory processes can also produce local destruction or at least simulate it on the x-ray film. This is particularly true for mycotic diseases of the paranasal sinuses, which may be misinterpreted on radiographs as a malignant process on the basis of real or presumptive destruction of the lateral wall of the nose.

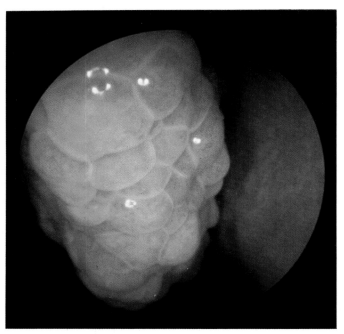

FIG 4–37.
Mucous membrane tuberculosis (in a case of open pulmonary tuberculosis). Right inferior turbinate.

The clinical symptoms are not helpful in distinguishing between invasive and chronic inflammatory processes, particularly in the early stages. A moderately symptomatic "chronic cold" may mask carcinoma of the lateral wall of the nose. Blood-stained secretions, on the other hand, should always be considered a serious indication of a hidden malignancy.

In neoplastic changes of the interior of the nose the surrounding mucosa frequently becomes edematous, and the ensuing, frequently significant polyp formation may completely obscure the underlying malignancy. For this reason, even in cases of apparent obvious polyps, every attempt should be made to carefully inspect all areas of the nose that can be reached with the endoscope. Granulating, lumpy changes should always raise suspicion of malignancy, particularly if they bleed easily on contact.

Inverted papillomas present their own, very special problems. Not uncommonly, inverting papillomas cannot be distinguished macroscopically from "normal" nasal polyps. Even the radiographic findings are confusing, unless there is already clear evidence of destruction and invasion. These patients have frequently undergone surgery for recurrent "typical" massive recurrent nasal polyposis, without any problems. Inverting papillomas do not always demonstrate the small granular to furrowed surfaces that are visible on the surgical specimen in Figure 4–38.

Our procedure in the case of an inverted papilloma is as follows. If the diagnosis is made only postoperatively from histologic examination of the surgical specimen and the patient was operated on for nasal polyposis, an ongoing thorough endoscopic follow-up is instituted. If the tumor was completely removed, there usually is no need for further therapy. Potential

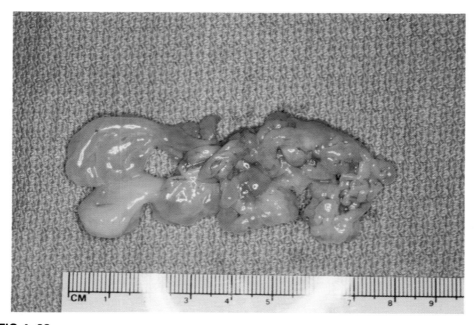

FIG 4–38.
Verrucous carcinoma. Cobblestone cauliflower-like texture on the surface of this "nasal polyp" is pathognomonic of verrucous carcinoma.

recurrences can be recognized and treated promptly. The rational basis for this approach is that histologically there should be no evidence for malignant degeneration in the removed neoplasm. If the diagnosis of an inverted papilloma is made preoperatively, further intervention depends on the size of the tumor. If endoscopically a relatively circumscribed base can be identified, we select an endoscopic surgical approach. If, however, the tumor shows evidence of destructive or invasive growth, there is no longer any indication for a primarily endoscopic intervention.

If there is malignant degeneration in the tumor, we use the endoscopic approach to obtain a biopsy specimen and to confirm the diagnosis. Resection of the tumor is performed by one of the proved external approaches, and the extent of the resection is determined by the findings.

5 Endoscopy of the Maxillary Sinus

INDICATIONS

Endoscopic examination of the maxillary sinus (sinuscopy) is a useful technique for evaluation of diseases affecting the interior of the maxillary sinus. When correctly and carefully performed, this minimally invasive procedure is well tolerated by the patient, with few risks and only the occasional minor complication. Maxillary sinus endoscopy is indicated when there is any suspicion of a specific or malignant disease process that requires a biopsy under direct vision. With this technique, samples can be taken for microbiologic analysis and culture (under anaerobic conditions, if necessary) with special equipment, and some foreign bodies can be removed from the sinus.

Maxillary sinuscopy is usually performed as a diagnostic procedure to correlate the patient's clinical symptoms with the radiographic findings, especially when the films cannot be clearly interpreted. In patients with symptomatic cysts, isolated polyps, or foreign bodies, the diagnostic approach is usually combined with therapeutic manipulation. Cysts may be punctured and their contents aspirated. Cysts walls, isolated polyps, and foreign bodies can be removed, and inspissated material can be aspirated and examined. In general, maxillary sinuscopy is the most accurate diagnostic technique for all disease processes within the lumen or that affect the mucosa of the maxillary sinus.

We are very conservative with maxillary sinuscopy in children, and rarely find an indication to perform this procedure in cases of inflammatory diseases of the sinuses in children. The exception is in children with antrochoanal polyps, in whom the maxillary portion of the polyp (which is usually cystic) is opened and removed via an endoscopic approach through the canine fossa.

Because of the degree of development of the child's dentition and the degree of pneumatization of the maxillary sinus, we do not perform maxillary sinuscopy via the canine fossa before the age of 9 years, to avoid potential damage to the dental germs. When maxillary sinuscopy is necessary in young children, we use an inferior meatal approach similar to that used for sinus irrigation. Specially designed narrow trocars that have an outer diameter of 3 mm and which can be used with the 2.7-mm endoscopes are available for this process.

Maxillary sinus endoscopy is not a routine component of a diagnostic or therapeutic endoscopic procedure.

INSTRUMENTATION

Relatively little instrumentation is needed to perform maxillary sinuscopy. The most important instrument is the trocar with its sleeve (Fig 5–1). The trocar has an outer diameter of 5 mm and a lumen through which the 4-mm diameter telescopes can pass. We prefer the shovel type of trocar sleeve over the blunt type. Various polyethylene catheters should be available to puncture cysts and for aspiration. A 10-mL syringe with a polyethylene catheter attached (which should be no longer than the trocar sheath) can be used to instill either saline solution to dissolve thick inspissated material in the sinus and facilitate its aspiration or topical vasoconstrictors in the event of mucosal bleeding. Additional topical anesthetics may also be administered by this route if required for biopsy purposes.

The biopsy forceps (Fig 5–2) are thin enough to pass through the trocar, and can be used to take biopsy specimens, to open and remove cysts, and to remove small polyps and inspissated material. These biopsy forceps can also be used to palpate the interior of the sinus, to determine the consistency of the mucosa, as well as to check for bony destruction in case of malignancy, and to help distinguish between polyps and edematous mucosa over the bony prominences of the sinus walls. The optical biopsy forceps enable the surgeon to perform a biopsy within the sinus under direct vision (Fig 5–3). Recently new aspiration forceps (Blakesley) have become available that can be inserted through the trocar.

A

B

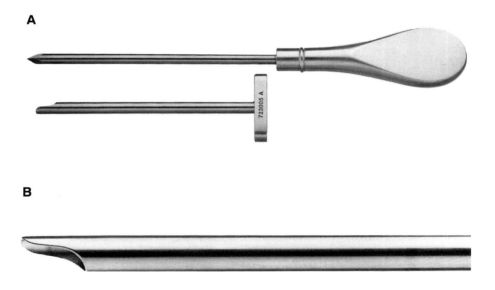

FIG 5–1.
A, trocar with sheath, outer diameter 5.0 mm. Note the shovel-like mouth of trocar sheath. **B,** detail of the trocar sheath. We prefer the shovel-shaped trocar sheath. It makes both manipulations within the maxillary sinus (displacement of cysts or polyps) and introduction into the middle meatus (e.g., careful introduction into a very tight middle meatus) easier.

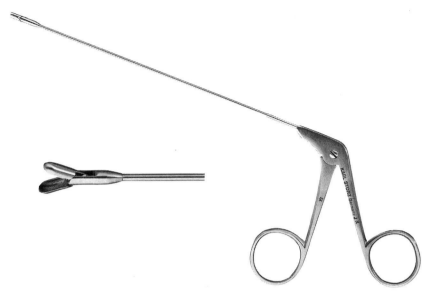

FIG 5–2.
A, biopsy forceps to be used through trocar sheath. **B,** close-up view of forceps mouth.

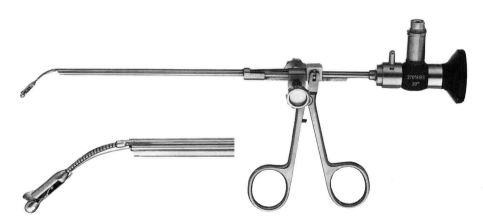

FIG 5–3.
A and **B,** optical biopsy forceps with 2.7 mm, 30-degree endoscope. For insertion through the trocar sheath, the flexible part of the forceps is maximally retracted. After insertion, the flexible forceps can be advanced gradually downward into the visual field of the 30-degree lens.

The ideal endoscope for the initial diagnostic examination of the maxillary sinus is the 4-mm 30-degree endoscope. This endoscope usually provides a clear view of most areas of the sinus, with the exception of its anterior wall. The area of the maxillary ostium is almost always visible with the 30-degree lens. With the addition of the 70- and 120-degree 4-mm endoscopes, even the most remote corners, as well as the anterior wall through which the maxillary sinus was entered, can be inspected. The 0-degree straight forward-viewing endoscope is useful for aiming the cannula directly at those areas where further manipulation is required.

TECHNIQUE

Except in children, maxillary sinuscopy is routinely performed with local anesthesia. The patient lies on his or her back on the table, with a firm and stable support under the head. We prefer this position to the sitting or reclining positions, which are less comfortable for the patient.

Initially a cotton pledget that has been soaked in a mixture (5:1) of 2% tetracaine (Pontocaine) and epinephrine 1:1,000 and well wrung out is placed into the oral vestibule above teeth 3 and 4 (canine and first premolar). Lidocaine (Xylocaine) spray may also be used for this purpose. After a few minutes the swab is removed and the canine fossa infiltrated through an 18-gauge needle with 4 to 5 mL of a 1% lidocaine solution containing epinephrine 1:200,000. The bony depression of the canine fossa can usually be easily palpated and identified. It is important that the local anesthetic reach the maxillary periosteum, and preferably some anesthetic should also be infiltrated near the infraorbital nerve and toward the piriform aperture of the nose.

After about 2 minutes of gentle massage performed to help spread the local anesthetic evenly through the soft tissues of the canine fossa, the trocar is inserted through the mucosa of the canine fossa. It is helpful for orientation if one finger rests at the inferior margin of the orbit. No incision is made in the mucosa. The tip of the trocar is inserted into the lateral aspect of the canine fossa high above the space between the roots of the canine and the first premolar inferolateral to the infraorbital foramen (Fig 5–4). First, with gentle rotation of the entire trocar the mucosa is pierced; then the orientation of the trocar in the lateral aspect of the canine fossa is reconfirmed. A constant to-and-fro rotating movement is applied to the trocar, which is slowly advanced through the anterior wall of the maxillary sinus.

The thickness of the anterior bony wall of the maxillary sinus varies among patients, and consequently the pressure to perforate this wall must be adapted to the individual. Sometimes the bone appears to be paper thin, and the trocar slips effortlessly into the maxillary sinus. In other patients the bone offers marked resistance, and considerable rotation pressure must be applied to penetrate the wall. When applying increased pressure, the surgeon must be prepared to stop immediately after the trocar has passed through the anterior bony wall to avoid damage to the posterior wall of the sinuses and to the structures within the sinus.

The surgeon should have studied the appropriate radiographs before the procedure to keep the dimensions and the topographic relations of the individual maxillary sinus in mind eye during insertion of the trocar. The trocar should be aimed toward the maxilloethmoidal angle (medial, posterosuperiorly located corner of the maxillary sinus). In this direction one usually will find the largest diameter of the sinus and minimize the risk of iatrogenic damage. In no circumstance should the trocar be aimed toward the floor of the orbit.

The piriform aperture and the bony medial wall of the sinus in the inferior meatus sometimes protrude much farther lateral than would be expected from the outer configuration of the nose (Fig 5–5). The bony margins of the piriform

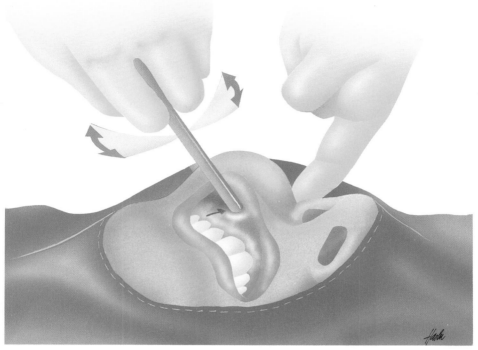

FIG 5–4.
Schematic drawing of the twisting, to-and-fro movement when the trocar is inserted. Note the index finger of the left hand palpating the inferior margin of the orbit. The tip of the trocar was pierced through the mucosa high in the oral vestibule in the projection of the line between teeth 3 and 4, well above their roots.

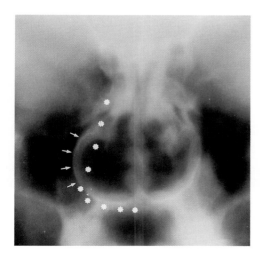

FIG 5–5.
Tomographic cut demonstrating a far laterally bulging medial wall of the maxillary sinus (*arrows*). The lateral contour of the soft parts of the outer nose is indicated by the line of asterisks.

aperture should therefore be identified by palpation before insertion of the trocar. Avoid inserting the trocar close to the piriform aperture, to avoid perforating the medial wall of the maxillary sinus and entering the inferior meatus of the nose.

With experience, the surgeon inserting the trocar through the anterior wall of the maxillary sinus should be able to identify the different phases of the perforation. First there is minimal resistance when sliding the trocar through the oral mucosa, which has been thickened by the injection of local anesthetic. This is followed by firm resistance when the tip of the trocar reaches the anterior bony wall of the maxillary sinus. One then identifies increasing resistance as the bone is drilled through during the to-and-fro twisting movement of the trocar. And finally there is a gradual decrease in resistance as the pointed tip of the trocar begins to enter the sinus. The trocar should be removed from the cannula only after the opening of the shovel of the cannula has been fully inserted into the lumen of the sinus. If when inserting the endoscope through the cannula one finds that only half of the trocar lip has entered the sinus, the trocar should be replaced inside the cannula and the puncture completed (Fig 5–6). The cannula should never be forced through the anterior wall without the trocar in place.

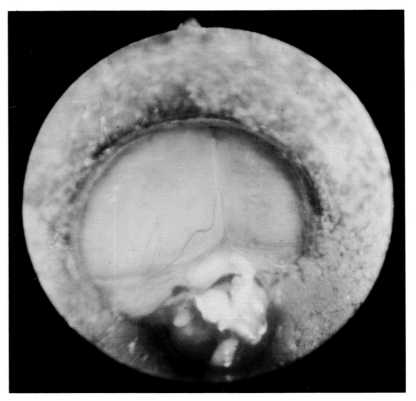

FIG 5–6.
In the left maxillary sinus, two cysts bulge into the trocar sheath inserted via the canine fossa. Note that the sheath has not yet completely entered the sinus and therefore needs to be advanced after reattachment of the trocar core, before any manipulations start.

Despite the bulky looking instruments, this procedure is usually well tolerated by the patient. Because of the infiltration of local anesthetic containing a vasoconstrictor, there is usually little bleeding.

The main advantage of this technique compared with the approach via the inferior nasal meatus is the wider range of mobility of the trocar sleeve. Without additional stress to the patient, the trocar sleeve can easily be rotated, and consequently all corners of the maxillary sinus may be inspected (Fig 5–7). This extra range of rotation is especially helpful when surgical manipulations are required within the sinus, because wherever one can point the cannula can be reached with instruments. Only when the bone of the anterior maxillary wall is excessively thick will the movement of the trocar sleeve be restricted. Pain may also restrict movement of the trocar sleeve if the initial puncture was performed too close to the dental roots.

Any mucosal bleeding within the sinus usually can be stopped by the appropriate instillation and aspiration of topical decongestants or vasoconstrictors through the trocar sleeve. When required, additional topical anesthetics can be instilled through the trocar before a biopsy or other manipulation is performed.

If a surgical endonasal procedure is planned and maxillary sinuscopy is also indicated, we always start with the sinuscopy. In some patients it is advisable to leave the trocar sleeve in situ after the maxillary sinuscopy until the surgery in the middle meatus has been completed and the natural maxillary ostium has been widened via the middle meatal approach. The widened ostium can then be checked from both sides. If during surgery difficulties arise in locating the natural ostium of the maxillary sinus from the middle meatus, direct

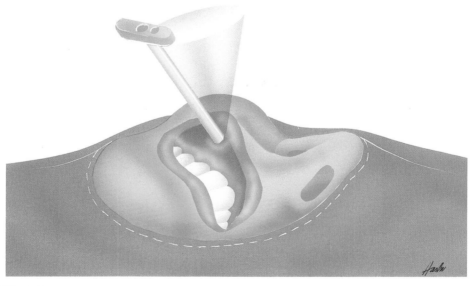

FIG 5–7.
Schematic drawing demonstrating the arc of rotation of the trocar sheath that can be used with this approach without discomfort for the patient.

visualization through the maxillary sinus toward the medial maxillary wall can be helpful (Fig 5–8). Moreover, an accessory ostium in the fontanelles of the middle meatus may be palpated through this route. Finally, in those cases where inspissated material must be removed from the sinus (e.g., fungal disease) or isolated polyps need to be resected, the trocar sleeve becomes a helpful instrument allowing the surgeon to manipulate in the maxillary sinus from both sides (Figs 5–9 and 5–10).

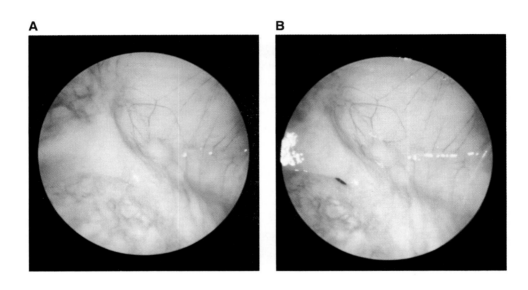

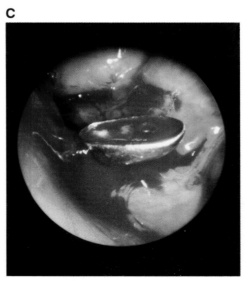

FIG 5–8.
A, left maxillary sinus, looking from the canine fossa toward the area of the natural ostium, which is blocked. **B,** during the Valsalva maneuver, the ostium opens a little bit and thus can be identified. **C,** under direct visual control, a bent spoon can be inserted via the middle meatus into the natural ostium and the latter consequently enlarged at the expense of the anterior fontanelle.

A

B

C

D

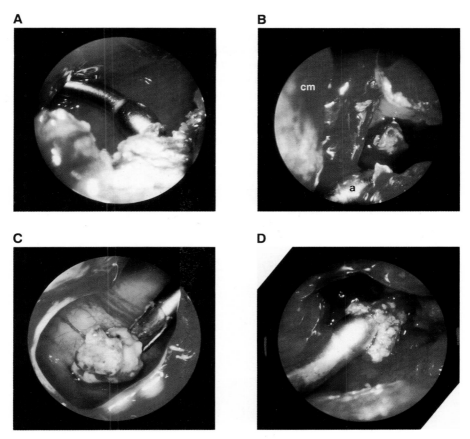

FIG 5–9.
A, a view into the maxillary sinus through the canine fossa. A right-angled suction tip has been introduced from the middle meatus through the enlarged maxillary sinus ostium, and additional fungal masses were removed. **B,** view into the maxillary sinus from the middle meatus through the enlarged window. There is still a cherry-sized fungal ball in the maxilloethmoid angle. *cm* = middle turbinate; *asp* = tip of aspirator. **C,** this fungal ball is pushed toward the maxillary sinus ostium with the trocar sheath. **D,** the suction tip picks up and removes the fungal ball.

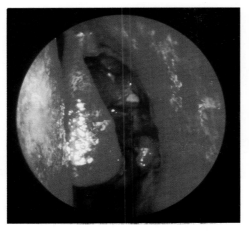

FIG 5–10.
The view into the middle meatus after completion of the surgical procedure. No packs are placed. The distance between the middle turbinate and the lateral wall of the nose is wide enough to prevent synechia.

Manipulation in the Maxillary Sinus

A biopsy is performed by aiming the trocar sleeve with the 0-degree endoscope in place toward the appropriate area. The trocar sleeve is then firmly held in place, the endoscope removed, the biopsy forceps inserted, and a specimen taken blindly. For the experienced surgeon this technique is faster and more effective than using the optical biopsy forceps. The same aiming technique can also be used to take specimens for culture.

To open maxillary sinus cysts, we use the following technique. The trocar sheath is directed toward the cyst and, if possible, pressed against the cyst wall so that it bulges into the lumen of the cannula (see Fig 5–6). Depending on the thickness of the cyst wall, we sometimes succeed in opening the cyst by twisting the cannula; otherwise, the tip of a polyethylene catheter is cut to a point (Fig 5–11), and with this harpoonlike instrument the cyst wall can usually be

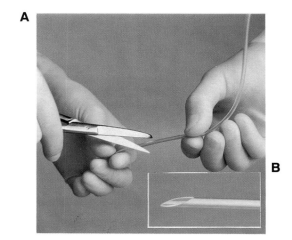

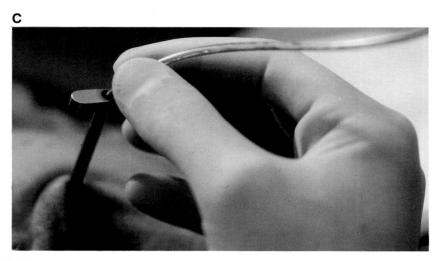

FIG 5–11.
A, a polyethylene catheter has been cut with scissors. **B,** the end is cut at an angle to form a point. **C,** the catheter is then inserted through the trocar sheath to puncture the cyst and aspirate its contents.

pierced. The cyst contents are then aspirated, and the cyst wall collapses. With this technique of aiming the cannula, under visual control, directly toward the cyst, multiple maxillary cysts can be opened sequentially. If the collapsed cyst walls cannot be aspirated, they can be grasped with the biopsy forceps and removed. Through the cannula, excellent optical control can be achieved (Fig 5–12). Only occasionally do we use the optical biopsy forceps (see Fig 5–3) to remove remnants of the cyst wall under direct vision, because the angulation that can be achieved with the flexible forceps is usually inadequate.

Foreign bodies, depending on their size and composition, can usually be removed through a maxillary sinuscopy trocar in many cases, as illustrated in Fig 5–13, extravasated root filling material was removed from a maxillary sinus. This material was too large to be transported through the natural ostium, but it was possible to shovel the debris onto the lip of the cannula and then

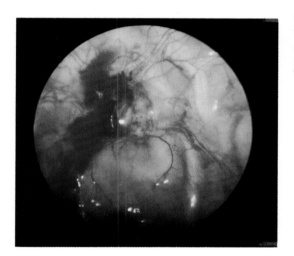

FIG 5–12.
View into the sinus after complete removal of the cyst. Only a minor mucosal lesion indicates the origin of the cyst.

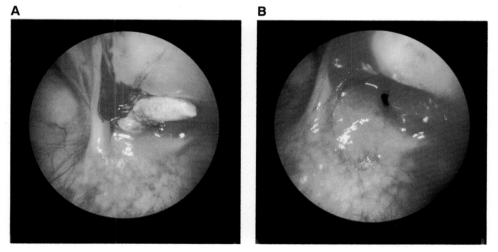

FIG 5–13.
A, dental filling material transported to the maxillary sinus ostium. This cylinder was too large to go through the ostium, so it remained and caused irritation. **B,** the extent of the irritation is visible after removal of the foreign body.

remove it with an aspirator. In other cases with larger foreign bodies, we attempt to break the material down into smaller portions, which can then be aspirated through the cannula. This technique, of course, is ineffective when the material is too hard to be split into smaller parts.

If the inspissated material is too viscous to be aspirated, it sometimes helps to instill a few drops of a mucolytic or saline solution and to wait for a few minutes before aspirating.

The diameter of the suction catheter should be small enough to always allow some air to pass into the maxillary sinus between the cannula and the suction catheter. If the suction catheter completely fills the lumen of the cannula, negative pressure will develop in the maxillary sinus if suction is applied when the sinus ostium is blocked. This can be very painful for the patient.

If there are isolated pedunculated (stalked) polyps on the walls of the sinus that are difficult to reach via the middle meatus, we proceed as follows. The stalk of the polyp can usually easily be cut or shaved off the sinus wall with the trocar sleeve, leaving the polyp free within the maxillary sinus. The polyp can then be pushed toward the widened maxillary sinus ostium (with the help of the trocar sleeve), where it is grasped with a suitable instrument and removed via the middle meatus.

In general, we do little surgery within the maxillary sinus. We do not consider diffuse polyposis of the maxillary sinus or even an empyema to be an indication for maxillary sinuscopy. We would not operate on an isolated asymptomatic maxillary sinus cyst as long as it does not block the ostium or radiographically is not suspicious for more serious disease. If endoscopic surgery is being performed on the lateral nasal wall and maxillary sinus cysts are present, we try to open the cysts during the same procedure.

At the conclusion of the diagnostic or therapeutic procedure, the trocar sleeve is pulled out of the sinus with the same twisting movement. The mucosal defect in the oral mucosa does not require a suture. The defect usually closes airtight within the next 2 days. During this period, patients are advised not to blow their nose, to avoid subcutaneous emphysema.

COMPLICATIONS

Maxillary sinuscopy is well tolerated by the majority of patients. Discomfort may be experienced by those patients who have had previous Caldwell-Luc procedures, because the scars in the area of the previous window through the canine fossa are usually more sensitive to pressure and pain. We have had surprisingly few problems with permanent dysesthesia or other irritations of the infraorbital nerve after maxillary sinuscopy. Occasionally patients complain of temporary numbness of the upper lip or the maxillary teeth on the side of the sinuscopy, but this usually disappears within a few days.

We have had only a handful of patients among thousands who complain of persisting dysesthesia attributable to irritation of the infraorbital nerve. In our experience, it is important to penetrate the anterior wall of the maxillary sinus as far laterally in the canine fossa as possible. In this area there are anastomotic branches between the sensory fibers of the rami buccales superiores of the facial nerve (the pes anserinus minor) and the infraorbital nerve. Consequently, a lesion to one nerve fiber in this area bears less risk of permanent sensory deficit.

More commonly we have seen emphysema of the soft tissues of the cheek when patients unintentionally blow their noses in the first few hours after the sinuscopy. None of these, however, has led to any persistent problem. The emphysema will resorb within a few days if the patient does not blow his or her nose. Depending on the individual situation, an oral antibiotic may be required in some of these cases. If maxillary sinuscopy is performed in cases of an acute sinusitis with empyema, there is a risk of infection of the soft tissues of the cheek. For this reason, we do not routinely perform maxillary sinus endoscopy.

Early in our experience, we found that after we had instilled antimycotic ointments and solutions into ethmoidal or maxillary sinus operative cavities (for cases of mycotic sinusitis) via the middle meatus on the first and second postoperative days, a number of patients developed painful and long-lasting granulomatous infiltrations of the soft tissues of the cheek. This apparently occurred because the antimycotic ointment reached the soft tissues of the cheek through the still patent trocar perforation in the canine fossa. Currently we postpone the instillation of antimycotic substances into the operative cavity until the fifth or seventh postoperative day, by which time the trocar perforation has sealed, thereby preventing the extravasation of ointment into the soft tissues of the cheek. Since we started this protocol we have not seen this complication. When in a noninvasive mycosis all of the fungal material has been removed, we do not use any antimycotic instillations.

When the trocar sheath is withdrawn from an infected maxillary sinus, care must be taken that no infectious material is "implanted" into the perforation channel, because this could lead to a sublabial abscess. The tip of the sheath must be cleansed by suction, and we prefer to keep a suction catheter inside the trocar as it is withdrawn.

There are several possibilities for "false passages." The lateral wall of the nose can bulge a surprising distance into the maxillary sinus, a configuration that cannot be predicted from the external shape of the nose. This creates the risk of a false passage into the inferior meatus. If the anterior wall of the maxillary sinus is perforated too far inferiorly, there is a risk of injury to the roots of teeth, particularly those of the canine and the first premolar. In children, care must be taken not to damage the dental germinal centers. The patient's radiographs should be carefully checked for unerupted teeth and for the dimensions of the maxillary sinus. This is why we normally do not use a canine fossa approach in patients younger than 9 years, depending on the development of the sinus (Figs 5–14 and 5–15).

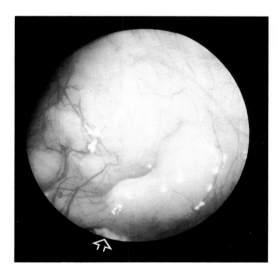

FIG 5–14.
Right maxillary sinus. Protrusion of the roots of second molar teeth through the alveolar recess. The mucosa appears normal. If the trocar sheath (*arrow*) is inserted too close to the maxillary sinus floor and advanced too far posteriorly, the tips of the dental roots might be injured in such a case.

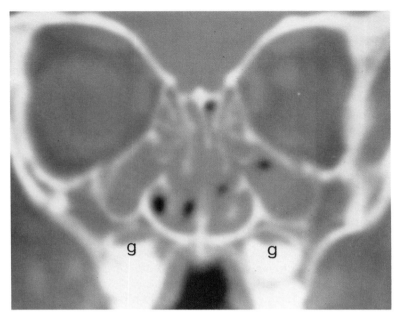

FIG 5–15.
CT scan of a 7-year-old boy with cystic fibrosis. The floor of the maxillary sinus is between 5 (*left side*) and 8 (*right side*) mm above the lowest level of the floor of the nose. *g* = dental germs in the alveolar recess contacting the floor of the maxillary sinus.

If excessive force is used when the trocar is inserted through the anterior wall (especially when the bone is thick and hard), breakthrough and damage to the structures of the posterior maxillary wall may result from failure to stop immediately after penetrating the anterior wall. Potentially one could enter the retromaxillary fossa and damage the structures therein, producing hemorrhage and risk for infection. We have not encountered damage to the posterior wall in our series of patients, but we believe that a careful technique is critical in avoiding such a problem.

We maintain that it is important that the patient lie on his or her back on a firm table, because this provides the best support to the head and allows the surgeon to aim and direct the trocar to the correct desired angle and position. If one uses shear force and does not insert the trocar with a twisting and rotating movement, the anterior wall of the maxillary sinus might infracture, and pieces of bone may be displaced into the maxillary sinus. In such circumstances, if the bony fragment is small and still adherent to normal mucosa, no further treatment is usually required. If, however, larger bony fragments without mucosal attachment are free in the lumen of the maxillary sinus and it is evident that they are too large to be transported out through the natural ostium, these splinters must be removed via an external approach.

Bleeding with maxillary sinuscopy is rare, and is usually the result of acute inflammation or tumors of the maxillary sinus. The few drops of blood caused by the trocar insertion usually allow for an elegant examination of the mucociliary transportation mechanism, because the blood-stained maxillary sinus mucus is transported toward the natural ostium (see Chapter 1).

ENDOSCOPIC FINDINGS

In this section some of the more clinically important and some unusual endoscopic findings in the maxillary sinus are discussed.

Symptomatic cysts are the most common indication for maxillary sinuscopy. It should be noted that the size of a maxillary cyst does not necessarily correlate with the severity of the symptoms that it produces.

Figure 5–16 shows a maxillary retention cyst that was smaller than a pea, yet produced chronic midfacial pain. This small cyst could not be demonstrated on plain films; however, tomography revealed the tiny cyst located on the canal of the right infraorbital nerve. Figure 5–17 shows the endoscopic appearance

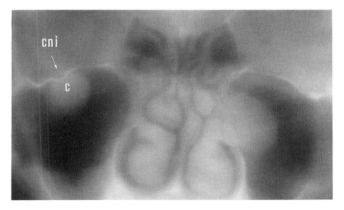

FIG 5–16.
Tomographic view of a maxillary retention cyst on the canal of the right infraorbital nerve. *cni* = infraorbital nerve canal; *c* = cyst.

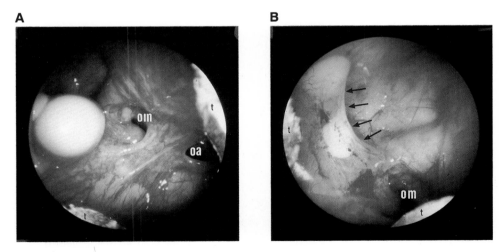

FIG 5–17.
A, endoscopic appearance of the cyst (see Fig 5–16) near the maxillary ostium and an accessory ostium. *om* = maxillary sinus ostium; *oa* = accessory ostium; *t* = trocar. **B,** after cyst removal, the course of the infraorbital nerve was visible *(arrows)*. *om* = maxillary sinus ostium; *t* = trocar.

of the yellowish white cyst located along the course of the infraorbital nerve on the roof of the maxillary sinus not far from the natural maxillary ostium. An incidental finding was an accessory ostium in the posterior fontanelle. After removal of the cyst through the trocar sleeve, the course of the infraorbital nerve was identified. The patient's midfacial pain disappeared after removal of the cyst.

Figure 5–18 demonstrates the endoscopic finding of a larger cyst that was present in the left maxillary sinus and that had originated from the area of the posterior nasal fontanelle. This larger cyst was easily removed through the trocar sleeve after having been punctured and its contents aspirated.

The patient in Figure 5–19 was to undergo an operation for anterior ethmoidal disease. His problems resulted in part from a large overpneumatized ethmoidal bulla. When performing maxillary sinuscopy to investigate the spherical "soft tissue" mass at the roof of the left maxillary sinus, we were surprised to find completely normal mucosa with no disease at the roof of the sinus. Because the tomograms had been performed only the day before the endoscopic surgery, it seemed unlikely that a cyst or a polyp had vanished in such a short time.

By accident, we were able to unveil the secret of this phenomenon. Time and again, we have seen balls of mucus up to 5 mm in diameter being transported over an apparently normal mucosa. Figure 5–20 shows a mucus ball at the roof of a right maxillary sinus inspected via the enlarged window in the middle meatus some weeks after surgery. The mucus ball in these cases consisted of a highly viscous but nonpurulent mucus. The sphere apparently results from the surface tension of either the thick mucus itself or the overlying gel layer of the "normal" mucus blanket. In any event, the adhesion between the normal mucous layer and the isolated ball of mucus must have been strong enough to prevent the mucus ball from dropping by gravity down to the floor of the sinus.

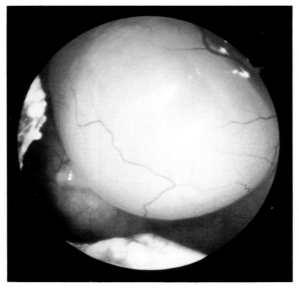

FIG 5–18.
Large cyst found within the left maxillary sinus.

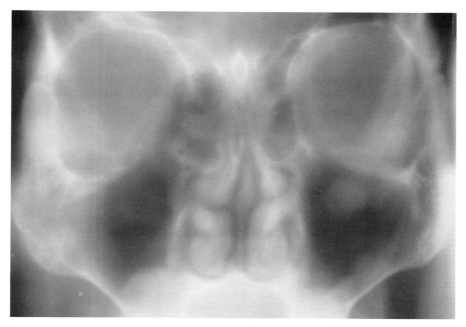

FIG 5–19.
Tomogram showing opacity at the roof of the maxillary sinus.

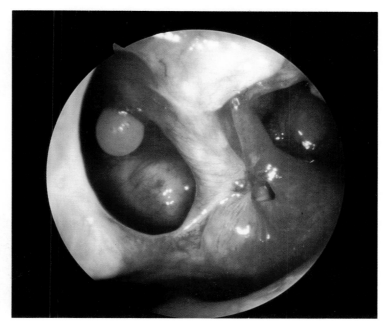

FIG 5–20.
Ball of mucus being transported along the roof of a right maxillary sinus.

Whether this phenomenon is the result of a localized abnormality of the mucosal glands or of some other pathologic process is unknown. So long as these mucus balls can be transported out of the sinus, they do not appear to have any pathologic significance.

The ability of the ciliary beat and the adhesive forces of the mucus layer to transport relatively heavy items upward to the natural ostium of the maxillary sinus is nicely demonstrated in Figure 5–13. A small metal cylinder of dental root filling material that had reached the maxillary sinus has been transported all the way up to the natural ostium. Because it was too large to pass through the ostium, it was retained there, causing irritation to the ostial mucosa. After removal of the foreign body through the trocar sleeve, the mucosal irritation around the ostium can be clearly seen (see Fig 5–13). This foreign body weighed 3.5 g!

Cysts in the maxillary sinus can originate from many areas. Retention cysts can arise from almost any area of the maxillary sinus mucosa. Cysts that result from dental problems are usually located on the floor of the maxillary sinus in the alveolar recess.

Not all cysts within the maxillary sinus necessarily arise from the sinus mucosa. Cysts and cystic polyps can expand into the maxillary sinus from the anterior ethmoidal sinus. For example, in Figure 5–21 the thin stalk of the cyst that has collapsed after being punctured can be seen clearly entering the right maxillary sinus through its natural ostium. Infundibular disease was present, and the stalk of the cyst was traced back to diseased mucosa in the hiatus semilunaris and the anterior face of the ethmoidal bulla.

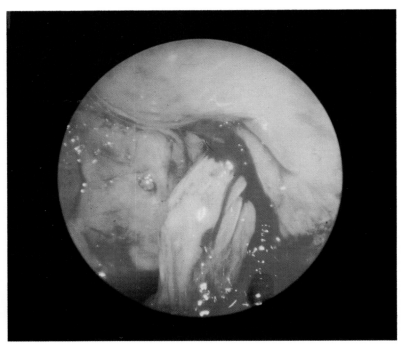

FIG 5–21.
Cystic polyps in the maxillary sinus.

The tomogram in Figure 5–22 shows a patient in whom root filling material was pressed into the maxillary sinus. The dentist's attempt to remove this material resulted in an oroantral fistula with a secondary maxillary sinusitis. This situation is shown in Figure 5–23, where a probe can be seen entering the left maxillary sinus through the fistula. The sinus mucosa is inflamed, and there is pus around food particles that have entered the sinus through the fistula.

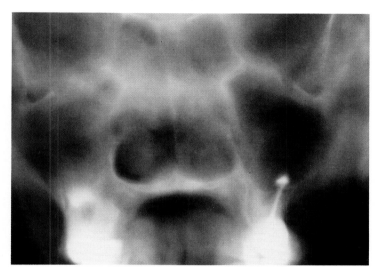

FIG 5–22.
Tomogram of a patient with dental filling material in the maxillary sinus.

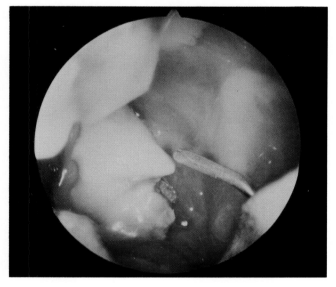

FIG 5–23.
Same patient as in Figure 5–22 viewed endoscopically revealed the oroantral fistula, as well as inflamed mucosa, a probe entering via the fistula, and pus-surrounded food particles.

Figure 5–24 shows an *Aspergillus fumigatus* fungal ball in a right maxillary sinus. There is currently no active inflammation. The fruiting heads of the *Aspergillus* can be seen on the surface of the fungal ball. There was one streak of whitish thickened secretion running from the floor of the sinus (not visible in this picture) to the natural ostium that contained fruiting heads and fungal spores running from the floor of the sinus (not visible in this picture) to the natural ostium. A second streak of mucus entered the maxillary sinus via an accessory ostium in the anterior fontanelle and was transported upward toward the natural ostium, where it left the sinus, only to enter again through the accessory ostium. This is an example of mucus recycling between an accessory ostium and the natural ostium.

A

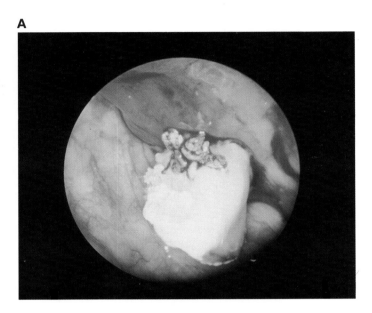

B

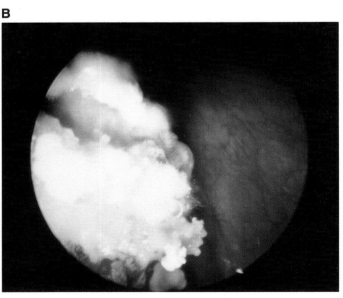

C

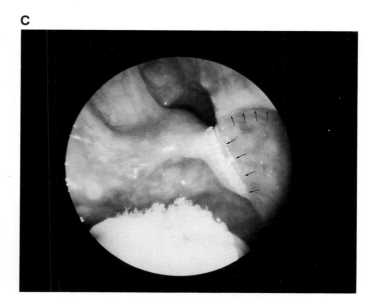

FIG 5–24.
A, note the cherry-sized fungal ball lying on top of the edematous mucosa on the floor of this right maxillary sinus. **B,** mycelia of the fungal growth are more clearly seen in this closer view. **C,** although the ostium of the maxillary sinus was patent, it was too small for the passage of the concretion. The transportation of spores and other fungal debris can be seen clearly traveling along the secretion pathways (*arrows*).

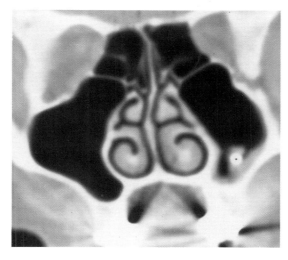

FIG 5–25.
Another patient with dental filling in the maxillary sinus has a CT scan that demonstrates the radiopaque material to be metal (M = 2,560).

Figure 5–25 demonstrates the computed tomography (CT) scan of another patient in whom dental root filling material has gone astray in a left maxillary sinus. The radiographic density measurement (2,560) clearly identifies the radiopaque material as metal. The mucosa around the foreign body appears to be swollen. The endoscopic findings are shown in Figure 5–26. Endoscopy was performed several weeks after the CT scan, when symptoms from the maxillary sinus developed. The mucosa is now extensively inflamed, and the root filling material that protruded into the sinus cavity is covered with pus.

The initial irritation of the sinus mucosa from dental filling materials is said to be caused by the disinfecting chemicals added to the material. In our experience, aberrant root filling material within a maxillary sinus predisposes to fungal sinusitis, and for this reason we recommend its removal even when the patient is free of symptoms.

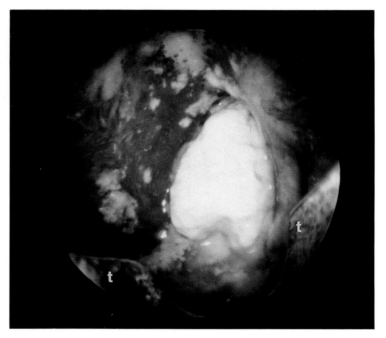

FIG 5–26.
A view into the left maxillary sinus of the same patient. The maxillary sinus also contained whitish masses characteristic of *Candida* mycosis. A carcinoma of the lateral wall of the nose was identified as the predisposing cause. *t* = trocar sleeve.

6 Indications and Contraindications for Endoscopic Surgery

The indications for endoscopic sinus surgery are derived from a combined assessment of the patient's history, the results of the endoscopic diagnostic examination, and the findings from the tomographic films. A surgical procedure is indicated only when it is justified by the patient's symptoms and when medical therapy is not successful or when the changes are such that medical therapy is doomed to failure.

Opacities on the radiographs without related clinical symptoms are an indication for further diagnostic exploration and evaluation in order not to miss a hidden malignancy. Once a malignancy has been excluded, no surgical procedure should be planned if the patient is experiencing no symptoms. In this situation, we discuss the findings with the patient and explain those symptoms that, for example, might someday be produced by large cysts of the maxillary sinus. The patient is informed that surgical intervention will be necessary only when and if these symptoms appear. Exceptions are mycoses, mucoceles, and other conditions that can be expected to produce problems sooner or later and thus may be indications for a surgical procedure, even in the absence of symptoms.

The most important and frequent indications for endoscopic sinus surgery in our patient population are summarized in Table 6–1, although this is by no means a complete list of all possible indications. We should emphasize those indications in which there seems to be no relationship between the patient's history and involvement of the paranasal sinuses, particularly when the plain

TABLE 6–1

Range of Indications for Functional Endoscopic Surgery

Polyposis	Eustachian tube problems
Obstructed nasal respiration	Postnasal drip
Recurrent and chronic sinusitis	Continuing complaints after Caldwell-Luc
Epiphora (tearing)	procedure or intranasal fenestration
Anosmia	procedures
Chronic headaches	As adjuvant therapy in allergies
Mucocele of any paranasal sinus	Sinubronchial syndrome
Retention cysts	Bronchial asthma
Mycoses (noninvasive)	Recurrent pharyngitis
Orbital complications of acute sinusitis	Some phonation disturbances
Septal spurs	Special cases of snoring

sinus radiographs are normal. In this context, headache of unknown cause, some eustachian tube problems, increased or pathologic secretions in the nasopharynx (postnasal drip), and tearing should be mentioned. Anosmia may be of rhinogenic origin without any rhinoscopic or plain radiographic basis. Some facial neuralgias may originate in the ethmoidal sinus, although these may also be related to such problems as deviation of the nasal septum. It is in these patients that high-quality conventional or computed tomograms (CT) are especially important.

It is not surprising that many patients undergo endoscopic sinus surgery for treatment of "nasal polyps." The mucosa of the ethmoidal sinus and other paranasal sinuses is limited in its response to inflammatory and other stimuli. Circumscribed swellings, edema, and ultimately polyp formation predominate. The formation of nasal polyps should be regarded as a nonspecific reaction of the mucous membranes to a variety of inflammatory, immunologic, allergic, chemical, toxic, thermal, or mechanical stimuli. It may be the result of the simultaneous influence of a number of these factors on localized or extensive areas of the mucous membranes, with a variety of stimuli producing a similar clinical morphologic appearance. Consequently, the diagnosis of nasal polyps is more of a description of the end result rather than a definition of the type or cause of a specific disease.

"Simple" nasal polyps should be distinguished from diffuse polypoid sinusitis on the basis of clinical appearance and behavior. Diffuse polypoid sinusitis is apparently the result of a generalized mucous membrane disease rather than a more or less circumscribed area of diseased mucous membrane (mucosal disease vs. diseased mucosa).

On the basis of the diagnostic information provided by the combination of the endoscopic examination and CT, one can obtain a large number of individual surgical indications that are more specific than could be expressed by the classic catchall term "sinusitis." In principle, many recurrent inflammatory diseases of the paranasal sinuses are the result of anatomic variations that require surgical correction and which can be corrected with the Messerklinger technique.

CONTRAINDICATIONS

The Messerklinger technique is not designed for the surgical approach to extensive, invasive procedures in the area of the paranasal sinuses or skull base. Extensive bony changes such as a broadly based osteoma are also not suitable for treatment with this technique. Coarse bony postinflammatory stenoses of the ostium of the frontal sinus are rare findings, which may stretch the usefulness of the endoscopic technique to its limits. Enlargement of the ostium of the frontal sinus after an osteitic process is not a suitable procedure for the instruments developed for the Messerklinger technique and cannot be performed with the patient under local anesthesia.

If the area of the frontal recess and the ostium of the frontal sinus can no longer be accurately identified from the nose because of scarring or ossification following previous surgery, a two-pronged approach is possible. Through a burr hole in the anterior wall of the frontal sinus (e.g., as in the Beck procedure), a 30- or 70-degree lens can be introduced into the frontal sinus, enabling the endonasal approach from the frontal recess to be visually controlled from above. In such cases of osteal stenosis or obstruction, we leave a polyethylene drain in place for 3 to 6 months after appropriate surgical enlargement of the ostium.

If in an orbital extension of an acute sinusitis there is even the slightest indication of an incipient central complication (e.g., meningitis, subperiosteal or epidural abscess, cavernous sinus thrombosis) or if there is evidence of osteitis or osteomyelitis of the frontal bone with sequestration, a primary endoscopic procedure according to the Messerklinger technique is contraindicated. The same holds true for orbital complications in which there is an acute visual or visual field loss or blindness. In these situations, and especially when there is sequestrum formation or an intracranial complication, we prefer a traditional, anterior approach.

In two rare cases we open the maxillary sinus through the canine fossa in inflammatory diseases:

1. Some mycoses, when the mycotic mass completely fills the maxillary sinus and cannot be broken up into smaller fragments or be satisfactorily removed via the middle meatus through an enlarged ostium, or when there is a suspicion of an invasive mycotic infection.
2. In some cases of previous radical maxillary sinus surgery, when the recess is scarred and compartmentalized and where it can no longer be reached and opened endoscopically with any degree of confidence.

ROLE OF ENDOSCOPE IN MEDICAL MANAGEMENT OF ACUTE SINUS INFECTIONS

The pathophysiologic mechanisms leading to an acute frontal or maxillary sinus infection have been discussed. It should be emphasized that most cases of acute sinusitis do not require surgical management.

However, the endoscope has a useful role in the medical management of an empyema of the frontal or maxillary sinus (Fig 6–1). In most cases of acute frontal sinusitis, even when there is already an obvious air-fluid level, the placement of epinephrine and tetracaine (Pontocaine) pledgets may decrease the swelling of the frontal recess, thereby allowing spontaneous drainage from the frontal sinus. Under endoscopic guidance, these pledgets can be placed with accuracy. With a slender alligator forceps or a bayonet forceps, the pledgets can be advanced with gentle pressure underneath the middle turbinate into the frontal recess, and left in place for 20 to 30 minutes. This form of therapy is repeated two to three times each day in addition to the administration of appropriate antibiotic and anti-inflammatory medical therapy. In this way even severe cases of acute sinusitis can be cured. It is most impressive to see the stream of pus that emerges from the engorged and inflamed nasal passages after the placement of a decongestant pledget into the ethmoid area, particularly into the frontal recess (see Fig 6–1). The endoscopist can usually see clearly where the source of the (secondary) frontal sinus disease is.

With this technique, we have not needed to use the Beck burr hole technique during the last 15 years for the treatment of acute frontal sinusitis.

In cases of acute recurrent or drug-resistant frontal sinus disease, we attempt to identify the underlying changes in the middle meatus and in the frontal recess by means of endoscopy and CT so that we may promote a cure

A

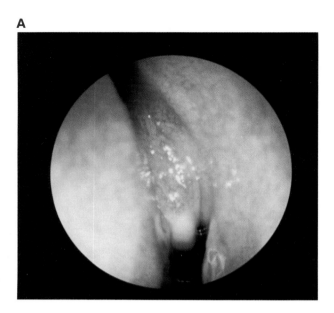

B

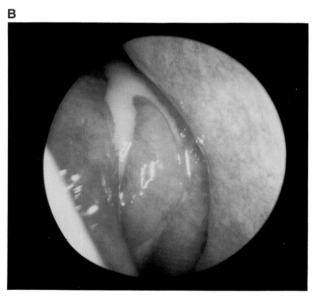

FIG 6–1.
A, this is the left middle meatus of a patient with pansinusitis. The uncinate process is folded sharply medially and is in close contact with the middle turbinate. No purulent secretions can be seen, even though the nose was sprayed with tetracaine and a vasoconstrictor. **B,** after the 15-minute application of a decongestant pledget directly into the middle meatus, a profuse flow of pus can be seen coming from the anterior ethmoidal sinus.

with the appropriate surgical intervention. The timing of this surgical intervention depends entirely on the clinical course of the disease. If there is no response to the conservative therapy described earlier, we endoscopically open the frontal recess after 2 to 3 days, provided there are no complications. If severe pain persists despite conservative therapy, we may intervene even sooner.

Frontal sinus surgery from the outside for inflammatory disease is usually required only for the reasons discussed (see Contraindications). Under no circumstances is an air-fluid level or an uncomplicated empyema sufficient indication for an external approach, and especially not for a radical procedure such as obliteration of the frontal sinus.

A similar goal-oriented local therapy is also useful in the treatment of acute maxillary sinusitis. We may perform an initial maxillary sinus puncture and irrigation through the inferior meatus even in acute primary sinusitis, depending on the clinical findings and the severity of the case. This is followed by placement of a local decongestant and anesthetic pledget into the middle meatus. This usually eliminates the need for serial punctures. By following this approach, we have not yet found a need to insert an indwelling catheter into the maxillary sinus.

In acute, purulent sinusitis accompanied by severe pain, it is advantageous to use not only a topical vasoconstrictor but also a topical anesthetic (e.g., 2% tetracaine). This provides symptomatic relief, particularly when the first insertion of a pledget produces only slight or transient improvement in drainage. It is always amazing to see the enormous amount of retained, purulent secretions that can emerge from the middle meatus and from the sinuses after a 20-minute application, and the great relief that the patient obtains from this simple and noninvasive procedure.

ENDOSCOPIC APPROACH TO CHRONIC HEADACHES AND SINUS DISEASE

Recurrent headaches can be frustrating for both the patient and the physician from whom treatment is expected. In general, the otorhinolaryngologist sees three different and distinct groups of patients with headache:

1. Those with headaches clearly resulting from sinus disease, such as in-flammatory disease, neoplasm, barotrauma, or another readily identifiable sinogenic cause.
2. Those with headaches that can be traced to nonsinus causes such as migraine, neuralgias, cervical spine disorders, abnormalities of blood pressure or other vascular disorders (ice cream headache), temporomandibular joint disease, ophthalmic refraction problems, glaucoma, and allergies.
3. Those whose problems are not clear and in whom there seems to be no overt indication of sinus disease. This group of patients can present a very rewarding challenge for the nasal endoscopist.

The typical triad of sinusitis symptoms includes nasal congestion or obstruction, the presence of abnormal secretions, and headache. The distribution of the headaches may be quite variable. Of 100 consecutive patients seen in our clinic with the diagnosis of acute or chronic sinusitis, 48 complained variably of headache as the predominant symptom. The typical pattern of possible sinugenic headaches is pain at the very top of the calvarium, sometimes together with a centrally located or bitemporal pain, indicating possible sphenoid or posterior ethmoid disease. Pain around the glabella, around the inner canthus, between or above the eyes, or intraorbitally suggests the presence of anterior ethmoidal sinus or frontal sinus disease.

Sinugenic headaches may also be experienced in the area of the temples, in the temporoparietal region, and in the occipital area. The pain may radiate from the forehead or the temples to the nuchal area or may circle the head like a tight band. The pain is usually characterized as "dull" and is accompanied by a feeling of pressure and fullness. In acute cases there may be pulsating pain, especially when the head is bent forward or when the patient is under physical stress.

These headaches may be the result of (1) constant intense mucosal contact, according to the concept of "referred pain"; (2) malventilation or nonventilation of the sinuses, with resulting hypoxia, or negative pressure; (3) pressure from proliferating polyps; or (4) epithelial lesions (or any combination thereof).

If only one symptom of the triad prevails clinically, we will still look for sinusitis if this symptom is congestion or suppurative rhinorrhea. If the symptom is headache alone and all results of our examination seem to be normal (routine sinus radiographs, anterior and posterior rhinoscopy, nasal endoscopy), we still consider the possibility of a sinus-related cause, especially when additional examinations by the ophthalmologist, dentist, internist, neurologist, and others reveal no pathologic findings and cervical spine radiographs, electroencephalographs, and CT scans of the brain are normal. Detection of disease in the narrow spaces of the lateral nasal wall hidden to casual examination and conventional radiographs is a challenging task for the endoscopist.

Through the use of the rigid nasal endoscope, the examiner may be able to identify relatively easily any underlying causes such as tumors, specific diseases such as sarcoidosis, and even high and posteriorly located septal spurs. It is well established that septal spurs or deviations contacting the turbinates may cause "contact" headaches, and the mechanisms of referred pain in lesions of the septal and turbinal mucosa have also been well demonstrated.

Endoscopic diagnostic techniques combined with CT enable the surgeon to discover disease otherwise hidden from the eye, the operating microscope, and conventional radiographs. Some of the typical and more frequent findings in patients with headache are listed in Table 6–2. Not all of these conditions should

---

TABLE 6–2

Frequent Endoscopic or CT Findings in Patients With Sinugenic Headaches

*Septal deviation or spurs
†Diseased agger nasi cells
†Diseased frontal recess

Uncinate process
†Medially bent, contacting middle turbinate
*Laterally bent
†Curved anteriorly (doubled middle turbinate)
*Fractures (trauma, iatrogenic)

Abnormalities of middle turbinate
†Concha bullosa (pneumatized middle turbinate)
*Paradoxically bent
*Bulging into lateral nasal wall

Ethmoidal bulla
‡Large, filling middle meatus
†Contact areas (especially polyps from turbinate sinus)
*Anterior growth, overlapping hiatus semilunaris
†Protruding from middle meatus
Combination of the above, resulting in obstruction of the frontal recess or of other parts of the middle meatus
   Isolated sphenoidal disease
* = rare finding; † = more frequent finding; ‡ = very frequent finding.

be considered a disease per se, but all are factors that can reduce the normally narrow spaces of the anterior ethmoidal sinus and give rise to areas of mucosal contact, secretion retention, and malventilation or infection of the larger sinuses or promote polypoid degeneration of the opposing mucosal surfaces. All of these conditions, even when minimal and circumscribed, may have one dominating clinical symptom: headache.

In Chapter 5 the endoscopic and CT findings are described in detail. At this point, we wish to emphasize the frequency of pathologic findings in the area of the ethmoidal bulla. The ethmoidal bulla may be pneumatized (enlarged) to such degree that it completely fills the sinus of the middle turbinate (the space in the convexity of the middle turbinate). This is one of the key findings in many patients with headache. The contact between bulla and turbinate can be extensive, almost like that of gauze packing of the middle meatus. It is important to recognize this condition on CT or conventional tomography, as it may be overlooked or read as normal, because there is normally no radiographic opacification of either of these structures in the case of contact headaches.

Some limited disease in the frontal recess and the infundibulum may cause severe symptoms and may even be clinically unrecognizable even with the endoscope. Diagnostically these are the cases in which CT and endoscopy complement each other. Time and again we have been able to identify relatively small polyps or cysts in the depths of the infundibulum as the underlying cause of headaches of many years standing.

The frontal sinus is a common source of headaches when it is malventilated or otherwise diseased. Because the area of the frontal recess is not always easily accessible with the endoscope, a combined diagnostic approach (CT and endoscopy) is critical. Similar symptoms may occur less commonly because of scarring or synechia in the middle meatal area after surgery, nasal packing, nasotracheal intubation, or nasogastric intubation.

UNUSUAL LESIONS

A number of more unusual lesions can cause sinugenic headaches. Isolated sphenoidal sinus lesions such as cysts, polyps, or mycotic infection can give rise to a more central headache. At endoscopy, a stream of pus or viscid mucus sometimes can be seen in the sphenoethmoidal recess, and sometimes it may not be possible to evaluate the sphenoidal sinus ostium directly. Sphenoidal sinus lesions may be recognized on a plain radiograph, but are better defined on CT scans.

The foramen rotundum with the second branch of the trigeminal nerve may lie in close relationship to the mucosa of the sphenoidal sinus in the event of extensive pneumatization. If the sinus is diseased, this may well affect the nerve and produce symptoms like those of trigeminal neuralgia. The vidian nerve may also lie in close relation to an extensively pneumatized sphenoidal sinus and thus be irritated in cases of sinus disease. With these possibilities in mind, we can expect on occasion to unearth the underlying cause of an allegedly "idiopathic" neuralgia, which then can be treated surgically with success.

When one or more of these possible causes of symptoms have been identified and medical therapy has failed, endoscopic surgery is indicated. If doubts about the indication exist, in some cases it may help to anesthetize the area of the suspected lesion (e.g., with cocaine or tetracaine) in the office in the same way as in the operating room, with cotton-tipped probes. If the patient is then free of headache or of the particular symptoms for the duration of the anesthesia, this may help the surgeon to make a decision regarding an operation.

The most impressive results are usually seen in patients in whom the predominant symptom has been headache and the underlying causes had been identified. Within a few hours of the endoscopic procedure the pain usually is gone, providing often dramatic relief despite the fact that reactive swelling, congestion, and mucorrhea may linger for several days after the procedure. For endoscopic surgeons, it is therefore one of the most challenging, yet rewarding, tasks to identify and treat causes that underlie allegedly non-sinus-related headaches.

Because the patient with a sinugenic headache may not have a typical history of sinus disease, we should investigate for underlying causes, such as nasal or sinus disease. Negative findings with anterior and posterior rhinoscopy, examination with the operating microscope, and conventional radiography do not rule out a nasal or sinus cause. Diagnostic endoscopy with rigid endoscopes in many cases allows detection of lesions hidden from the unaided eye or even from the operating microscope, although endoscopy will also sometimes miss disease in particular locations even if repeatedly carried out at intervals. Only the combination of diagnostic endoscopy with CT provides the maximum information, with one modality enhancing the accuracy of the other.

Because significant symptoms can sometimes be caused by relatively small lesions, attention in examining imaging studies should not be focused exclusively on opacifications or soft tissue masses in the sinuses or the lateral nasal wall but on the identification of areas of possible stenoses and mucosal contact areas, such as the frequent finding of a middle meatus completely packed by an extensively pneumatized ethmoidal bulla. This finding alone was frequently the explanation for severe headaches and a feeling of nasal obstruction.

The rhinologist should view the CT scans jointly with the radiologist and explain what kinds of changes and abnormalities are being searched for that may be of clinical importance. After identification of these underlying processes, functional endoscopic surgery with usually minimal procedures can often provide dramatic symptom relief that may continue for months and years.

7 Advantages of Local Anesthesia

The advantages of local anesthesia are obvious. In most cases local anesthesia provides excellent hemostasis and thus excellent visibility during the surgical procedure. This is practically never the case when general anesthesia is used. Local anesthesia makes it easier to distinguish healthy mucosa from diseased mucosa, to recognize anatomic narrowings, and to remove them carefully with the least radical procedure. This results in more rapid wound healing and less stress on the patient. With few exceptions, packing is not required in patients operated on under local anesthesia.

The risks of local anesthesia are less than those for general anesthesia, and even older patients at cardiac risk can usually be operated on without any problem. Intraoperative pain is an important early warning that contributes greatly to the avoidance of injury to the roof of the ethmoidal sinus, the orbit, and the optic nerve. Another important feature is that local anesthesia forces the surgeon to exert the greatest care and to proceed with as little trauma as possible. Even the well-sedated patient will not tolerate roughness under local anesthesia. The postoperative recovery time is clearly shorter after local anesthesia. Even after a total sphenoethmoidectomy, most patients can be up and about after 2 to 3 hours, take nourishment, and breathe through the nose.

Except in children, almost all of our endoscopic procedures are performed using topical and infiltration anesthesia in the premedicated, sedated patient. *General anesthesia should be reserved only for exceptional cases.* Whenever possible, we try to convince the patient of the advantages of local anesthesia. It is our conviction, supported by our clinical experience, that the Messerklinger technique *should not be performed with the patient under general anesthesia.*

PREOPERATIVE PREPARATIONS

As with any operation that will be performed using local anesthesia and for which the patient's understanding and cooperation are important, the purpose and nature of the endoscopic nasal procedure must be clearly explained. The indications, purpose, and expectations of the procedure have usually been discussed at the time of the diagnostic endoscopy. Tomograms or computed tomography (CT) scans are helpful in showing the relationship between the diseased ethmoidal sinus and the other paranasal sinuses and for pointing out the potential technical difficulties and risks that are inherent because of the topographic proximity of the neighboring structures. These relationships can be best demonstrated to the patient on the coronal CT images.

139

It usually comforts the patient to know the steps and sequence of the procedure as well as its approximate duration, because the patient will be a conscious participant. We inform the patient that after premedication has been administered, he or she will become very drowsy but not asleep, and consequently will be aware of most of the events taking place.

Patients are informed that although they will be aware that their nose is being operated on, they should not feel pain. Some minor bleeding is inevitable, but the loss of blood is usually slight and should not affect the patient in any way. The patient should always be sufficiently awake to tell the surgeon of the need to expectorate. Patients should always indicate promptly if they do not feel well, become nauseated, or feel faint. Patients should be made to feel like a participant in the procedure rather than helpless.

Before the procedure, we show the patient the cotton pledgets and explain their purpose and how long they will remain in the nose. We tell the patient that the pledgets will feel cool on introduction and that they may initially generate a feeling of slight pressure or discomfort. The patient is told that the subsequent injection of a local anesthetic may also generate a feeling of pressure or tension and that if a few drops of anesthetic reach the pharynx they can safely be swallowed. We also warn the patient about the sensation of pressure in the nostrils that may be produced by the surgical instruments. It is particularly important to allay the patient's anxiety about the cracking and sometimes snapping noises and the sensations that occur when the cellular septa and other bony structures of the ethmoidal sinus are removed.

Usually, apprehension about the procedure can be largely alleviated in most patients and their full cooperation obtained. Once the premedication has been administered, the patient should not be distracted by unnecessary questions or extraneous noises.

PREMEDICATION FOR LOCAL ANESTHESIA

A number of suitable premedications are available that can be used for procedures under topical and local anesthesia. The choice of agent is determined by the preference of the surgeon and the anesthesiologist, taking into account the individual requirements of the patient. The premedication administered should provide sedation, analgesia, and anxiolysis.

The surgical requirements that must be met by the anesthesiologist ordering the premedication are that the patient remain in contact, respond, and be able to follow simple commands, (e.g., swallow, spit, turn the head toward the surgeon). Furthermore, *the swallowing and cough reflexes must be preserved.* If the sedation is too profound and the surgeon loses contact with the patient, more problems are generated than resolved.

Our most commonly used and most satisfactory premedication consists of meperidine (pethidine hydrochloride) as a narcoleptic analgesic and promethazine both for sedation and as an antiemetic. Our standard dose for a healthy 50-year-old adult weighing 70 kg is 100 mg meperidine and 50 mg promethazine, given intramuscularly, 30 to 45 minutes preoperatively.

We do not use atropine for premedication, because the resultant dryness of the mouth is unpleasant for the patient and the decrease in secretions is of little, if any, benefit for surgical procedures in the nose.

The patient is brought to the operating room 10 minutes before the start of surgery, and the pledgets are placed in the nasal cavity. Respiration and circulation are monitored. An intravenous infusion is started even before the premedication is given, if possible on the patient's left side so that it remains accessible without disturbing the surgeon.

PATIENT POSITIONING

The head of the supine patient is slightly extended and turned to face the surgeon, who sits on the patient's right side. The surgeon's legs should fit under the table, approximately at the level of the patient's neck. In elderly patients it is sometimes necessary to support the head when decreased mobility of the cervical spine no longer permits a completely flat, supine position. We do not like the semirecumbent position (with the head and trunk slightly elevated) because this position makes it more difficult for the surgeon to assume a fully relaxed posture and also makes it much more difficult for the surgeon to visualize the frontal recess. The frontal recess can usually be easily examined by slightly hyperextending the patient's head. Figure 7–1 shows our standard setup.

Close to the surgeon on his or her left side is a small table that holds the endoscope and its handle, a storage vessel half filled with saline solution and

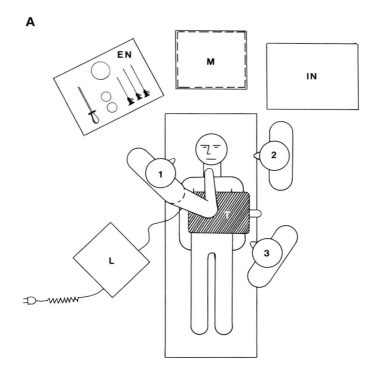

FIG 7–1.
A, this schematic representation shows the position of the patient for functional endoscopic sinus surgery using topical and local infiltration anesthesia. *1* = surgeon; *2* = scrub nurse; *3* = assistant; *L* = light source; *EN* = movable table with endoscope and accessories; *M* = video monitor, alternate location for light source; *IN* = movable instrument table; *T* = Mayo stand to hold suction tips and other equipment and serve as an armrest for the surgeon.

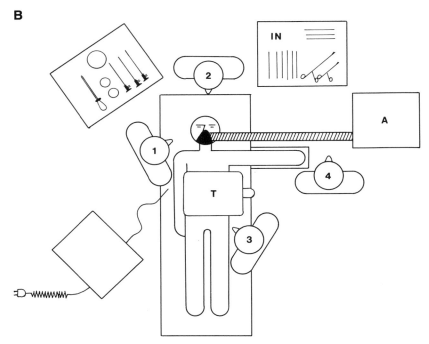

FIG 7–1. (cont.).
B, this illustration shows the position of the patient and the arrangement of equipment for an endoscopic sinus surgical procedure to be performed using general anesthesia. *1* = surgeon; *2* = scrub nurse; *3* = assistant; *4* = anesthesiologist; *T* = Mayo stand for instruments and armrest; *IN* = movable instrument table; *A* = anesthesia machine and its connections.

lined with absorbent cotton, antifogging solution, cotton pledgets, and epinephrine and tetracaine for topical anesthesia.

The surgeon changes and cleans the endoscopes and applies the antifogging solution to the lens. Arm rests on the chair are advantageous to prevent fatigue. The left elbow may also rest on the endoscope table. A Mayo stand on which the right elbow may rest is placed over the patient's chest (as for microlaryngoscopy).

The scrub nurse sits or stands at the patient's left side, across from the surgeon. Another assistant stands at the level of the patient's knees, on either the left or right side. This assistant hands the suction tip to the surgeon. The handing and changing of instruments must be performed smoothly so that the surgeon's eyes need not leave the endoscope. Frequent change from the eyepiece to room light can be very distracting. It should be noted that in this setup no instrument is ever passed across the face of the patient. This prevents injury if an instrument is accidentally dropped.

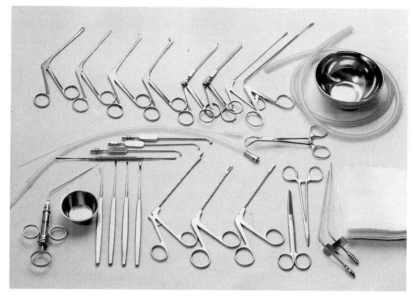

FIG 7–2.
Standard instruments for endoscopic procedures. *Bottom left:* 2-mL O-ring syringe with a septum needle for local anesthesia. A detailed description of the instruments can be found in the Appendix.

Endoscopic ethmoid surgery is not a particularly sterile procedure, because the inside of the nose cannot be sterilized. After cleansing the patient's face, a drape with a hole is placed over the face, leaving the mouth and nose free. The hole is wide enough to permit access to the eyes, if necessary.

The patient is covered with a sterile sheet. The nurse removes the required instruments from a sterile container just before the procedure and lays them out on the instrument table (Fig 7–2). The endoscopes are sterilized in gluteraldehyde solution, washed, dried, and covered with a sterile towel on the endoscope table.

It is especially important that the tomograms are displayed in the operating room so that the surgeon can see them by simply raising his or her eyes from the patient. Even after the most thorough preoperative study of the tomograms, the surgeon frequently encounters situations where review provides important information. This is even more important if several patients are scheduled one after the other, and provides additional safety for both patient and surgeon.

ADMINISTRATION OF TOPICAL AND INFILTRATION ANESTHETIC

For topical anesthesia and vasoconstriction of the mucous membranes, we use a mixture (4–5:1) of 2% tetracaine and epinephrine 1:1,000. This mixture is prepared in a small metal cup into which we place a number of small (1 by 1 cm) cotton balls, each having a ligature tail. These cotton pledgets are more convenient to use than standard neurosurgical sponges, because they are more absorbent and more easily molded. They are also easier to introduce into the recesses and corners of the common and middle meatus.

It is particularly important that the pledgets be completely wrung out before their introduction into the nose and after they have been soaked in the tetracaine-epinephrine solution. The pledget must not be dripping wet when applied to the mucosa. This gives us the best guarantee that only a minimal amount of tetracaine and epinephrine comes into contact with the mucosa. With careful attention to this principle, we have used this technique in several thousand patients without a single serious complication or side effect from either the tetracaine or the epinephrine. In older patients with hypertension, coronary artery disease, or cardiac arrhythmias, the surgeon should consult with an internist and the anesthesiologist to determine if tetracaine and epinephrine can safely be used.

The pledgets are introduced with bayonet forceps. Ideally they should be advanced to the entrance of the middle meatus, although this is not always possible because of the presence of a disease process. Regardless of the extent of the proposed procedure, an attempt should be made in each case to fill the entire nasal cavity with the pledgets. We usually push the first pledget to the end of the middle turbinate, both below and medial to it. We then place pledgets into the sphenoethmoidal areas and fill the space anteriorly from this point between the septum and the middle turbinate after having placed several pledgets into the middle meatus itself. It is important that the pledgets come into direct contact with the mucosa at the attachment of the middle turbinate along the lateral wall of the nose, the mucosa over the uncinate process, and in the area of the agger nasi. The anterior third of the nose is then loosely packed with pledgets all the way to the vestibule.

Under no circumstances should the mucous membrane be traumatized or injured during the placement of the pledgets. If rough handling causes even minimal bleeding, for example, in the area of the septum or of the lateral wall anterior to the middle turbinate, this bleeding can become a very real nuisance for the duration of the procedure and transform an ordinarily simple procedure into a troublesome and difficult operation. The pledgets must be placed very carefully and without any force; blood stains on the pledgets on removal indicate that these guidelines were not followed.

Cocaine (5% or 10%) may be used as a topical anesthetic instead of tetracaine and epinephrine. The excellent anesthesia provided by tetracaine, combined with the good vasoconstriction produced by epinephrine, and the total absence of side effects when used with the technique just described, has in our hands obviated the need for any other topical anesthetic.

The pledgets are left in place for at least 10 minutes, then removed from the operative side first, by carefully pulling on the suture attached to the pledget. The tetracaine-epinephrine mixture in the small cup is preserved in the event additional anesthesia is needed during the procedure.

For infiltration anesthesia we use 1% lidocaine with epinephrine 1:200,000. The injection is made under endoscopic guidance with a three-ring syringe and a special septal needle (see Fig 7–2). The typical injection sites under the mucosa of the uncinate process are shown in Figure 7–3. The technique of infiltration is the same as in septoplasty. The needle is introduced under the mucosa, and the solution is injected until the mucosa is slightly elevated from its base. This is readily indicated by mucosal blanching. Because in most cases the procedure begins with an incision into the ethmoidal infundibulum, 1 to 1.5 mL lidocaine is injected at three or four injection points. The most important points are in the area of the insertion of the middle turbinate, because the terminal branches of the anterior ethmoidal artery and nerve, proceeding from above, pass on to the middle turbinate and the agger nasi. It is also important to infiltrate the attachment of the uncinate process to the inferior turbinate, because if the ostium of the maxillary sinus must be enlarged, the area of the fontanelles may be exposed to considerable pressure by the instruments.

The number of injection sites should be kept to a minimum to avoid the possibility of oozing from the puncture sites. Great care must be exercised when introducing the needle so as to not injure the more anterior areas of the mucous membranes. The mucosa may be very thin over the nasal septum and also over the uncinate process, and thus it may be difficult to introduce the needle under the mucous membrane and elevate it with the injected solution. If the bone in the area of the uncinate process is very thin or absent, the needle may inadvertently be advanced into the infundibulum and the injected solution enter the nasopharynx. The patient should be advised of this possibility and informed that small amounts of the anesthetic solution can be swallowed without harm.

Only rarely is more than 1 to 1.5 mL lidocaine required to anesthetize each side. Under no circumstances should so much solution be injected under the mucous membrane of the uncinate that it distorts the contours of the uncinate itself or balloons the mucosa and obscures the view into the middle meatus. If this happens, it can be very difficult for the surgeon to find the proper location for the incision through the uncinate process.

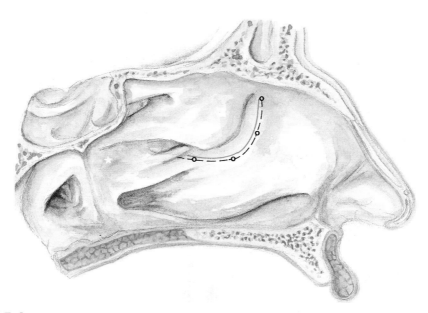

FIG 7–3.
Semischematic representation showing the injection sites for local anesthesia along the anterior insertion of the uncinate process. The anterior outline of the uncinate process is marked with a *red line*. The number of injections should be kept to a minimum, and the injections should always be made 2 to 3 mm from the insertion of the uncinate process under the mucous membrane (*o*, along the *broken line; arrows* indicate direction of infiltration). A *star* marks the area of the palatine foramen, where an additional injection may be made, if needed. NOTE: the middle turbinate is very short and small in this illustration (this corresponds to the skull cross-section used in Chapter 2). As a result, the uncinate process appears to extend far beyond the turbinate anteriorly and inferiorly. In the majority of cases, the insertion of the uncinate process runs parallel to the projection of the outline of the head of the turbinate onto the lateral wall of the nose (see Chapter 2).

Occasionally it is helpful to bend the tip of the needle to the right or left, particularly when one is trying to reach the posteroinferior end of a far lateral uncinate across a medially protruding middle turbinate. After injection of local anesthetic, it is advisable to wait 1 to 2 minutes before beginning the operation. During this period the points of injection may be gently compressed with the tip of the aspirator to prevent oozing.

If the procedure includes opening of a concha bullosa, injections are performed in a similar fashion under the mucosa of the head of the middle turbinate and along its inferior free margin toward the rear. If the entire middle turbinate is pneumatized, resection of the lateral lamella may present increased hazards, and the surgeon must remember that he or she may be operating perilously close to the sphenopalatine foramen and to the vessels and nerves that emerge from it. It is therefore particularly important to provide thorough anesthesia in the area of the end of the turbinate.

It is a source of constant amazement to us that in most cases it is possible to work in the area of the sphenoidal sinus without any additional anesthesia if the mucosa of the uncinate process was infiltrated really well.

If the patient reports pain during the operation, we use tetracaine-epinephrine–soaked pledgets to repack the surgical field loosely. This is most likely to occur when there is scarring from a previous procedure or in the presence of an acute inflammatory process.

The most pain-sensitive areas are the posterior end of the middle turbinate, close to the sphenopalatine foramen, and the inferior edge of the ostium of the maxillary sinus. Pain in the area of the roof of the ethmoidal sinus suggests the proximity of the anterior ethmoidal nerve and is an important warning signal.

We have no experience with transorbital block of the anterior and posterior ethmoidal nerves, and we perform a sphenopalatine block only rarely.

ENDOSCOPIC PROCEDURES USING GENERAL ANESTHESIA

General anesthesia should be reserved solely for the exceptional case and used only by the very experienced surgeon. Obviously, general anesthesia is required when operating on children. We are extremely conservative in assessing indications for endoscopic sinus surgery in children.

We will consider general anesthesia in adults when there is extensive scarring from previous surgery, if surgical revision of scarred and compartmentalized maxillary sinuses is necessary, or if osteitic changes or scars preclude local anesthesia for an approach to the frontal sinus. The incidence of general anesthesia in our patient population is less than 5% of all procedures. Even hypotensive general anesthesia does not provide as bloodless a field as local anesthesia. Posthypotensive rebound hypertension makes packing necessary more frequently.

When general anesthesia must be used, the nose should be prepared in the same way as for local anesthesia except that phenylephrine is used instead of epinephrine as an additive to pontocaine.

Even in the hands of an experienced surgeon, the amount of blood lost when general anesthesia is used can be five to 12 times as much as with local anesthesia (150–360 mL vs. <35 mL). In more than 6,000 endoscopic sinus surgeries performed with the patient under local anesthesia, blood transfusion was required in only one patient, because of massive blood loss.

8 Surgical Operative Technique

SURGICAL PRINCIPLES

Although total sphenoethmoidectomy can be performed with the Messerklinger technique, one of the major advantages of this technique is that because of the initial and precise diagnostic evaluation of the disease (even in severe cases), such extensive resection is only rarely necessary. On the basis of a step-by-step advance into the ethmoidal sinus, which is always targeted toward the patient's specific pathologic condition, the surgeon can usually identify and differentiate severe pathologic mucosal changes in the ethmoidal and sphenoidal areas from collateral edema, which requires no surgical removal.

Accurate diagnosis remains the keystone of the Messerklinger technique, even during the surgical procedure. Because most diseases of the paranasal sinuses originate in or depend on the ethmoidal sinus, the surgical procedure is focused on this area. Even in those cases with massive involvement of the frontal or maxillary sinuses, correction of the ethmoidal disease usually results in recovery of the larger sinuses within a few weeks, even though these sinuses have not been touched. In most cases, the ostium of the frontal sinus does not need to be touched, and fenestration of the maxillary sinus into the inferior meatus is not necessary. When required, the natural ostium of the maxillary sinus in the middle meatus can be enlarged at the expense of the adjacent anterior or posterior fontanelles. An enlarged natural maxillary ostium is much less likely to become stenotic than a fenestration into the maxillary sinus through the inferior meatus (inferior meatal antrostomy).

Every attempt should be made to achieve the desired results with the least traumatic procedure, to spare the patient from unnecessary "routine" radical procedures. This is facilitated by using a tissue-sparing and mucosa-preserving minimally invasive surgical technique targeted toward the specific pathologic condition and by the use of special instruments. The enormous regenerative potential of even massively diseased mucosa is always impressive.

The goal of the surgical procedure is not the creation of a large, smooth cavity connecting all of the paranasal sinuses, but to remove the obstructing, anatomic variations and to resect only the most severely diseased mucosa in these key locations. The mucosal lining should be preserved wherever possible. *Under no circumstances should extensive bony surfaces be denuded of their mucosal covering*, because this will increase the chance of postoperative osteitis. It is also not necessary to remove remnants of bony walls or septa with a diamond drill.

The Messerklinger technique cannot provide a surgical cure for all inflammatory paranasal sinus disease. In some polypoid paranasal sinus diseases none of the currently available surgical techniques can provide a definitive cure. Because, however, in these cases even radical surgical procedures do not assure a better long-term result, we feel confident in using the Messerklinger technique, which produces at the least similar results with much less morbidity and less intraoperative and postoperative stress for the patient.

HANDLING AND MANIPULATION OF SURGICAL INSTRUMENTS

Endoscopic surgery is primarily a one-handed procedure in which the instruments are introduced alongside and parallel to the endoscope. One of the surgeon's hands, usually the left, holds and controls the endoscope while the other hand manages the instruments and the suction tip (Fig. 8–1). Although initially this one-handedness may appear to be a handicap, the experienced surgeon will not notice this to be a problem, and the initial learning difficulties are more than compensated for by the remarkable clarity of the endoscopic

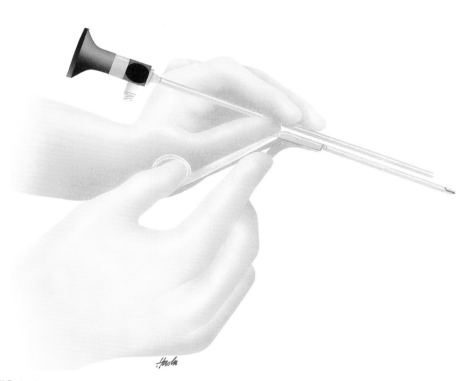

FIG 8–1.
Typical position of the hands in endoscopic surgery. For details, see text.

image, the outstanding depth perception, and the ability to move the instruments and the endoscope freely within the nasal cavity (Fig. 8–2). The mobility of the endoscope provides an excellent and almost three-dimensional spatial sensation that permits outstanding orientation, which can be enhanced by the surgeon's ability to look around corners by using a variety of angled lenses.

Insertion and manipulation of the endoscope, which is held like a pencil with three fingers (see Fig 8–1) can be made easier by the use of special sheathlike handles. These handles also help to compensate for the rotational force of the light cable, the observer side arm, or a television camera. With these special handles, the angled lenses can be more easily rotated around their long axis without the danger of losing the view and without the surgeon feeling cramped. Nasal specula or other holding devices are not required for either diagnostic or surgical procedures.

As shown in Figure 8–1, the endoscope is held in the middle of its shaft with the thumb, index, and middle fingers. The little finger and the edge of the left hand are rested very gently on the bridge of the patient's nose or cheek to help support and guide the endoscope. The endoscope is always introduced into the nasal vestibule under direct vision. This technique prevents incidental injury and avoids the nasal hairs, which may become coated with debris, mucus, or bloody secretions, and keeps the lens free from dirt and deposits. It is not usually necessary to cut the hairs in the nasal vestibule.

The introduction of the 30-degree telescope requires some skill; introduction of the 70-degree telescope requires considerable skill because it no longer permits a forward view along the long axis of the scope. The surgeon should use

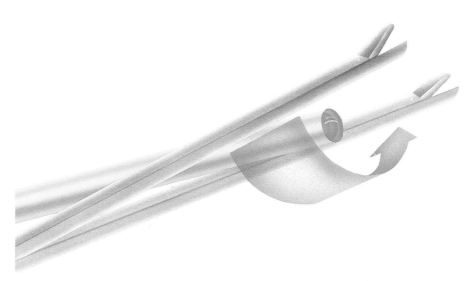

FIG 8–2.
Range of motion of the instrument around the endoscope.

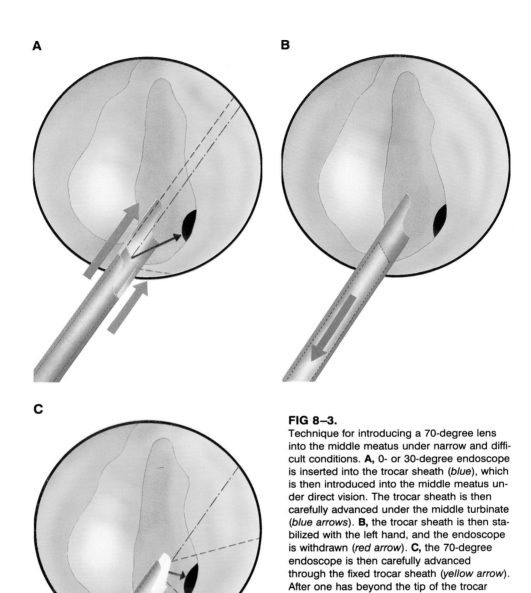

FIG 8–3.
Technique for introducing a 70-degree lens into the middle meatus under narrow and difficult conditions. **A,** 0- or 30-degree endoscope is inserted into the trocar sheath (*blue*), which is then introduced into the middle meatus under direct vision. The trocar sheath is then carefully advanced under the middle turbinate (*blue arrows*). **B,** the trocar sheath is then stabilized with the left hand, and the endoscope is withdrawn (*red arrow*). **C,** the 70-degree endoscope is then carefully advanced through the fixed trocar sheath (*yellow arrow*). After one has beyond the tip of the trocar sheath, an unimpeded view can be obtained of the target structure (in this case a look at and through the maxillary ostium).

the trocar sleeve to assist in the insertion of the 70-degree telescope (Fig 8–3). This is accomplished by first advancing the trocar sheath to the desired depth with the 0-degree telescope. The trocar sleeve is then held in position while the 0-degree lens is removed from the trocar sheath. The 70-degree telescope is then inserted into the sleeve.

A right-handed surgeon should always introduce the surgical instruments along the right side or underneath the scope (as shown in Figs 8–1 and 8–2), to assure the greatest mobility of the instrument without obstructing the surgeon.

As an instrument is introduced into the nasal cavity, it should always be advanced parallel to the axis of the endoscope, using the shaft of the endoscope as a guide. This is the best way to avoid accidental damage to the skin of the nasal vestibule and unnecessary injury to the mucosa of the anterior nasal passages. We recommend that the left eye be used as the guiding eye for the endoscope, allowing the right eye to be used to control the introduction of the operating instruments into the nose. To avoid injury, the surgeon should introduce all scissors and forceps in the *closed position.*

When one is changing instruments, it is advisable to take the guide eye away from the scope or to open the right eye so that the new instrument can be introduced under direct vision, thereby preventing accidental injury. With experience, the surgeon may become able to introduce instruments blindly by advancing them alongside the endoscope and guiding them into the nasal vestibule with the fingers of the left (scope-holding) hand. All change of instruments should be accomplished expeditiously and carefully but without undue haste.

The guiding principle of atraumatic surgery must be kept in mind at all times, because even the smallest mucosal laceration may cause enough bleeding to make the rest of the procedure extremely difficult. The same care should be devoted to the introduction of instruments in the nose as is used in middle ear surgery.

Because of the clarity of the optical image and the wide-angle effect of the nasal endoscope, there is an initial temptation to get as close as possible to the target area. During endoscopic sinus surgery, especially when the posterior ethmoidal or sphenoidal sinus must be reached, this can result in the formation of a tunnel or channel; although the individual details are extremely clear, the general overview is lost. This increases the risk of the surgeon losing depth perception and underestimating the depth of penetration into the nose. The endoscope should always remain as far as possible behind the instrument so that the anatomic landmarks necessary for proper orientation are always in view. Even when the surgical procedure involves the middle meatus, it is not always necessary to enter it with the endoscope.

The anterior insertion of the middle turbinate into the lateral nasal wall is the most important landmark for judging the depth of entry into the nose and the angle of the advancing instrument relative to the base of the skull and the lamina cribrosa. This is of critical importance when precise identification of the anatomic structures is no longer possible because of the extent of the disease (e.g., diffuse or recurrent polyposis).

The following procedure has proved helpful to us in providing a rough estimate of the depth of penetration into the nasal cavity. The index finger is placed on the shaft of the instrument at the level of the anterior nasal spine when the tip of the instrument is inside the nasal cavity. All of our suction tips are marked in centimeters; therefore, the depth of an intranasal instrument can be determined by laying the aspirator alongside the instrument inside the nose. It is also useful to check the position and the angle of the endoscope and of the instruments and their relationship to the base of the skull and the orbits by taking the eye away from the lens and looking at the setup from outside. This technique is useful in providing a rough orientation, but it can never replace precise visual identification of the anatomic landmarks.

The computed tomography (CT) scan also provides the surgeon with an excellent method of determining all of the important distances preoperatively. The most important distances and angles are those between the anterior nasal spine and the frontal recess, the roof of the ethmoidal sinus, the basal lamella, and the anterior wall of sphenoidal sinus.

With practice, the surgeon should gain an excellent feel for the spatial relationships by the relative motion of the endoscope and the instrument or by the simultaneous advancement and retraction of both. When one is working in the ethmoidal sinus, this freedom to change the direction of the view and of the approach, combined with the superb visibility provided by the nasal endoscope, gives this technique a definite advantage over the operating microscope.

Initially one may encounter some difficulty in avoiding contact between the lens of the endoscope and the mucosa or with secretions or blood. Such contact requires frequent withdrawal, cleaning, and reintroduction of the endoscope. The suction tip should always be introduced without suction until the tip appears in view through the endoscope, to avoid blood being drawn from the depth of the field, not only into the suction tip but also onto the lens of the endoscope.

When endoscopes are switched during the procedure, the endoscopes that are not in use should be immersed in a cotton-lined container of warm sterile saline solution. This prevents damage to the lens and the drying of blood and secretions on the lens. Before each introduction, the lens is treated with antifog solution, which is not wiped off but is left as a thin layer on the lens. The excess solution is usually lost during the passage through the vibrissae.

If, during a procedure, it becomes necessary to enter the middle meatus with the endoscope, and if the entrance to the middle meatus is very narrow, the instrument or a more slender suction tip can be used to carefully displace the middle turbinate medially, thereby allowing the endoscope to be introduced into the meatus. At the least, a good view can be obtained with this maneuver. When this is done, great care must be exercised not to injure the mucous membrane of the head of the middle turbinate.

We do not use the commercially available, suction-irrigation endoscopes, because they are too bulky. Entry into the middle meatus with these instruments is frequently impossible without injuring the head of the turbinate. In addition, the use of irrigation in the prone patient whose airway is not intubated is not possible, because the irrigating solution will run directly into the pharynx.

SURGICAL TECHNIQUE

In this section, the individual steps of functional endoscopic sinus surgery are illustrated on a cadaver. The steps shown are not necessarily routine, but include all steps that are technically possible with the endoscopic approach. Although the Messerklinger technique is suitable for the performance of a total sphenoethmoidectomy, the general idea is to avoid such routine radical procedures.

The preferred endoscope for the surgical procedure is the 0-degree (straight forward viewing) instrument. The 30- or 70-degree nasal endoscopes are used only in special situations, such as when the frontal recess is involved, when the natural ostium of the maxillary sinus is enlarged, or in procedures within the maxillary sinus.

The 0-degree nasal endoscope has many significant advantages, especially for the less experienced endoscopist. It is the only endoscope in which the axis along which the surgeon looks, corresponds exactly to the direction of its shaft, that is, the long axis of the instrument (Fig 8–4). When using a rigid endoscope, the beginner instinctively feels that the endoscope points in the direction of the image seen and that the instrument used is also located along the same axis. This is true only for the 0-degree nasal endoscope. Even a slight angulation, as with the 30-degree lens, can confuse the beginner and make anatomic and topographic orientation difficult. This is particularly true when the anatomic landmarks have been destroyed by the disease process or removed during a procedure.

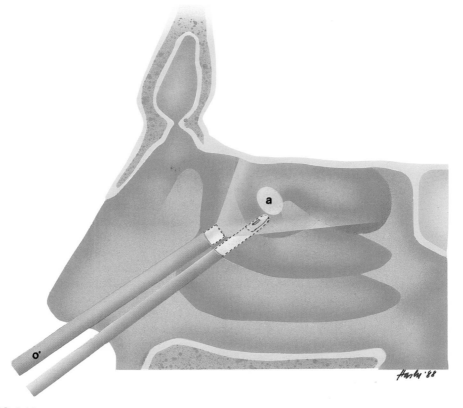

FIG 8–4.
Only with the 0-degree endoscope does the instrument point exactly in the same direction as the shaft of the endoscope and in the same direction as the view seen (*a*).

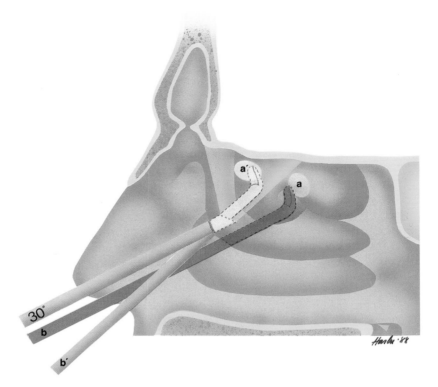

FIG 8–5.
Even with a 30-degree endoscope, one no longer looks in the direction in which the instrument points
(*a*), but depending on the orientation of the lens, [in this case anterocranially (*a´*)]. As a result, the
beginner may suffer from the misconception that he or she is working with the instrument in the same
direction in which the endoscope points (*a, b*). The surgeon is actually working at a considerable angle
from this direction because of the angulation of the endoscope lens (*a´, b´*). The angled lenses should
be used only after the key anatomic landmarks (roof of the ethmoid, anterior ethmoidal artery, etc.) have
been unmistakably identified.

The angle between the endoscope and the surgical instrument cannot be
appreciated by looking through the endoscope. As shown in Figure 8–5, the
surgeon will have the impression that the instrument is moving along the long
axis of the endoscope, in other words, that the action is occurring at the basal
lamella of the middle turbinate, when in fact the roof of the ethmoidal sinus has
already been reached. For this reason, we strongly urge all beginners in
endoscopic procedures to use the 0-degree endoscope as much as possible for
all of the surgical steps and to use the angled endoscopes only for the few
specific indications just given, and even then only after the important
topographic landmarks have been identified.

Figure 8–6 shows the starting position in a right nasal cavity. The 0-degree
nasal endoscope has been introduced through the naris, passed through the
nasal vestibule, and advanced 1.5 cm anterior to the insertion of the middle
turbinate without touching the septum or the lateral nasal wall. The endoscope
allows a direct view of the front of the middle turbinate, its insertion into the
lateral wall of the nose, and at the anterior aspect of the middle meatus. The free
posterior margin of the uncinate process, and behind it a portion of the anterior
surface of the ethmoidal bulla, can be seen.

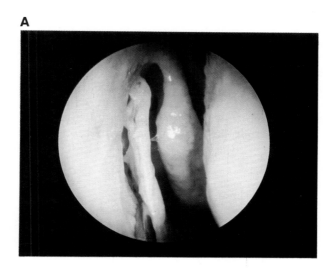

A

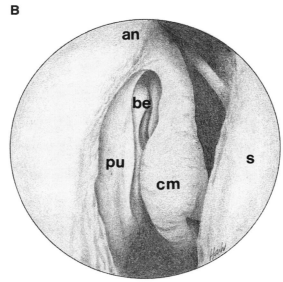

B

FIG 8–6.
A, view through a 0-degree endoscope into a right middle meatus. For a more detailed description, see the text. **B,** schematic drawing of **A,** *cm* = middle turbinate; *pu* = uncinate process; *be* = ethmoidal bulla; *an* = agger nasi; *s* = septum.

Resection of Uncinate Process (Infundibulotomy)

Because most sinus disease involves the anterior part of the ethmoidal sinus, the first step in most operations consists of opening the ethmoidal infundibulum by resecting the uncinate process. The medial wall of the ethmoidal infundibulum is formed by the thin bony uncinate process and its mucous membrane covering. The uncinate process is resected by inserting a curved knife blade (sickle knife) carefully into the uncinate process just below the insertion of the middle turbinate. The insertion of the uncinate process on the lateral wall of the nose is then transected in a convex arch from anterosuperior to posteroinferior. In this process, the tip of the sickle knife usually does not extend more than 3 or 4 mm through the uncinate process into the ethmoidal infundibulum. It is of the utmost importance that the knife be advanced through the uncinate process at a shallow angle (i.e., in a plane parallel to the medial wall of the orbit). We

A

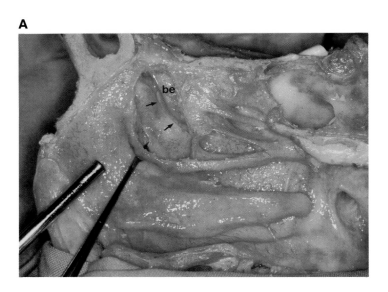

B

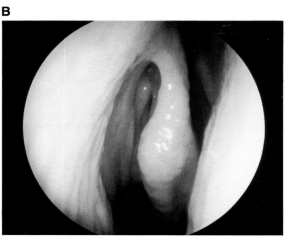

FIG 8–7.
A, right lateral nasal wall. The middle turbinate has been fenestrated so that the underlying structures can be seen. *Arrows* indicate the free posterior margin of the uncinate process. The hiatus semilunaris is located between the arrows and the anterior surface of the ethmoidal bulla. In this case, the bulla lamella extends to the skull base (*white arrow*) and separates the frontal recess from a potential lateral sinus. The sickle knife cuts around the anterior insertion of the uncinate process. **B,** endoscopic view of the same situation. The uncinate process was incised from above downward with the sickle knife. Note the shallow angle of the blade to the lateral nasal wall (to avoid penetrating the lamina papyracea).

always attempt to hold the handle of the sickle knife parallel to the lateral wall of the nose after its tip has penetrated the uncinate process. Under no circumstances should the sickle knife project so far laterally that it injures the lamina papyracea of the orbit.

It is always desirable to know before surgery the precise width of the ethmoidal infundibulum (i.e., the distance between the uncinate process and the lamina papyracea). If the infundibulum is very narrow or even atelectatic, the sickle knife must not point too far laterally at the point of insertion, and the incision should not be deep, because injury to the orbit may occur. In these cases, stepwise resection of the uncinate process in segments from back to front, as described earlier, has proved successful.

In Figures 8–7 and 8–8, a window has been cut into the middle turbinate so that the subsequent surgical steps can be demonstrated from the medial side.

A

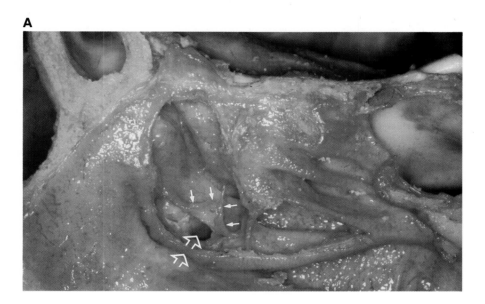

B

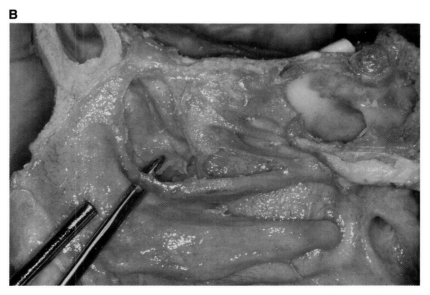

C

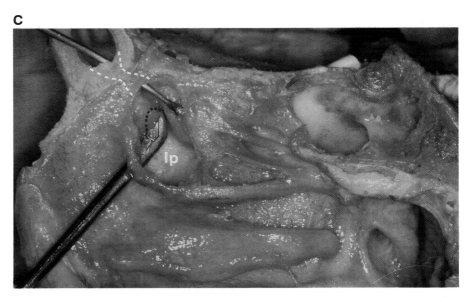

FIG 8–8.
A, view through the fenestrated middle turbinate. The anterior insertion of the uncinate process has been incised and displaced medially and superiorly (*small arrows*). The ostium of the maxillary sinus, hidden on the floor of the ethmoidal infundibulum, can now be plainly seen (*open arrows*). **B,** resection of the uncinate process. For a detailed description, see the text. **C,** after resection of the inferior two thirds of the uncinate process, one can see the lamina papyracea just above the ostium of the maxillary sinus. Note in this specimen how the ethmoidal infundibulum terminates superiorly in a blind pouch (the recessus terminalis). This happens because the uncinate process deviates laterally and inserts onto the lamina papyracea. The tip of the upward angled forceps dips into the recessus terminalis. The outline of the recessus terminalis is marked with *black dots.* A sound has been placed through the ostium of the frontal sinus, into the frontal recess. The *broken white line* shows the outline of the floor of the frontal sinus, with its funnel-shaped constriction toward the ostium of the frontal sinus and the adjacent, also funnel-shaped, enlargement of the frontal recess. The resulting hourglass configuration is evident. *lp* = lamina papyracea.

The uncinate process is then carefully displaced medially so that the surgeon can look directly into the ethmoidal infundibulum (Fig 8–9). The anterior wall of the ethmoidal bulla can be seen at the bottom, and any pathologic changes in this area can be identified.

The superior insertion of the uncinate process is then carefully grasped with a Blakesly-Weil forceps, without injuring the adjacent middle turbinate, and the bony insertion of the uncinate process is separated from the lateral nasal wall with a twisting motion of the forceps. The inferior insertion of the uncinate process is grasped with the Blakesly-Weil forceps and separated with a similar twisting motion so that the uncinate process can be removed in its entirety.

After the uncinate process has been circumferentially incised, it should not be simply pulled out with the forceps, because this can lead to uncontrolled tearing of the mucous membranes. This may occur particularly at the insertion of the middle turbinate, and leads to troublesome hemorrhage and the creation of opposing raw wound surfaces (e.g., between the lateral wall of the nose and the lateral surface of the turbinate). Even a few drops of blood in this area can make inspection of the frontal recess difficult.

A

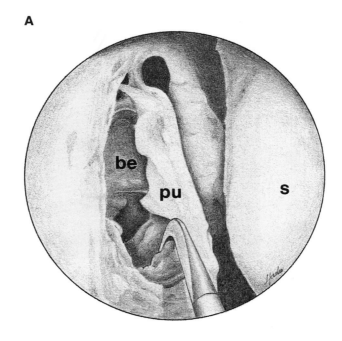

B

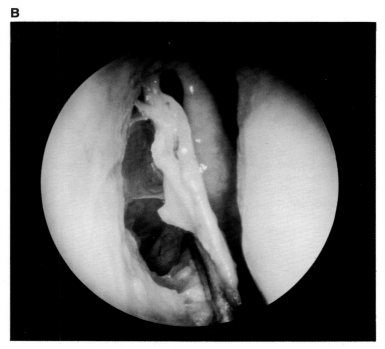

FIG 8–9.
A, endoscopic appearance after the uncinate process has been incised. The uncinate process is pushed medially with the sickle knife so that an unrestricted view is gained through the ethmoidal infundibulum to the anterior surface of the ethmoidal bulla. **B,** drawing of the endoscopic situation. *be* = ethmoidal bulla; *pu* = uncinate process; *s* = septum.

A

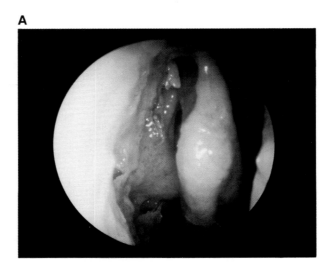

B

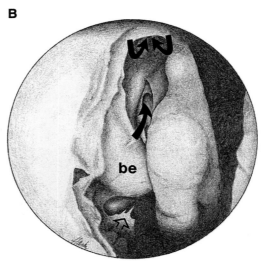

FIG 8–10.
A, endoscopic view after the major portion of the uncinate process has been removed. **B,** schematic drawing. There are a few small remnants of the uncinate (*open arrow*) covering the ostium of the maxillary sinus. The ethmoidal bulla is now exposed. The path to the lateral sinus (*single arrow*) posterosuperiorly through the hiatus semilunaris is medial to the bulla. The path to the frontal recess is now open anterosuperiorly (*curved arrows*). The frontal recess can be explored without resecting the bulla. *be* = ethmoidal bulla.

Figure 8–10 shows the endoscopic appearance after the uncinate process has been resected. The wide passage made into the anterior ethmoidal sinus can be seen clearly. The ethmoidal infundibulum no longer exists, because its medial wall (the uncinate process) has been removed. The anterior surface of the ethmoidal bulla limits the view posteriorly. Remnants of the insertion of the uncinate process can still be seen superiorly and inferiorly. These remnants can be removed if indicated by the pathologic changes present.

The anterior insertion of the uncinate process into the lateral wall of the nose cannot always be clearly identified. Occasionally the uncinate process can be identified by careful palpation. The anterior line of insertion of the uncinate process in many cases follows the projection of the anterior edge of the middle turbinate on the lateral wall of the nose. This is not a reliable landmark. When in doubt, it is safer to begin the resection at the posterior edge of the uncinate process, because this can almost always be clearly identified, and to resect the uncinate process anteriorly from this point by removing strips.

Depending on the disease, the uncinate process may consist of very solid bone or may have been thinned by inflammation or polyp formation to such extent that it is almost nonexistent. In this case there is practically no resistance to the sickle knife, and the "uncinate process" consists of only a double layer of mucous membrane.

Depending on the extent and location of the disease within the ethmoidal sinus, the surgical steps described may prove sufficient. The infundibulum has been opened, it can easily be inspected, and the surgeon can then determine if further procedures in the area of the frontal recess or the ostium of the maxillary sinus are required.

The ostium of the maxillary sinus frequently becomes visible after the uncinate process has been resected. If the ostium cannot be seen after resection of the uncinate process, it either is closed by diseased mucous membrane or may be hidden behind a posteroinferior remnant of the uncinate process. Such remnant can usually be identified by palpation with a small, angled spoon and then removed. Location of the maxillary sinus ostium may be facilitated by pressing on the lateral nasal wall with an instrument in the region of the anterior or posterior fontanelle. The appearance of small bloody bubbles may indicate the location of the natural ostium.

If the frontal sinus is involved, after the uncinate process has been resected the way is open to the frontal recess. If on the basis of the preoperative examination and tomogram or as a result of the intraoperative findings it becomes apparent that the ethmoidal bulla is also involved or that the resection must proceed to the posterior ethmoidal sinus or even to the sphenoidal sinus, these steps should be performed before the frontal recess is opened. This prevents even minimal bleeding, which can flow backward with gravity from the frontal recess into the posterior ethmoidal or sphenoid sinus and complicate the surgical procedure in these areas.

Tips for Identification of Site for Incision of Uncinate Process

Usually the anterior insertion of the uncinate process follows roughly the projection of the anterior free margin of the middle turbinate onto the lateral wall of the nose. There is frequently a small sulcus on the lateral wall of the nose at the insertion of the uncinate process. Posterior to this point the uncinate process can be readily incised. By palpation with an instrument, the uncinate process can frequently be indented and observed to spring back medially. This "movable" part of the uncinate can then be resected at a flat angle.

The safest method, however, is to identify the uncinate process at its free, posterior margin and, in case of doubt, to resect it in strips from the back anteriorly with a curved blade or a reverse biting punch forceps. When one is attempting to identify the insertion of the uncinate process, the mucosa at the insertion or of the agger nasi should never be injured with the curved blade. This will only cause unnecessary bleeding, which can make the rest of the procedure most difficult, and ultimately lead to granulation tissue and scar and synechia formation that may constrict the entrance of the middle meatus. When the agger nasi is extensively pneumatized, the bony lamella of the uncinate process may extend into the bony, medial wall of the agger nasi.

Resection of Ethmoidal Bulla (Anterior Ethmoidectomy)

If the ethmoidal bulla or the space between the medial wall of the bulla and the lateral surface of the middle turbinate (turbinate sinus) is diseased, the next step is resection of the ethmoidal bulla (Fig 8–11). Resection of the bulla is also indicated when a healthy bulla is so large that it completely fills the turbinate sinus, when it has extensive contact with the middle turbinate, or when the bulla extends anteriorly and overlaps the hiatus semilunaris, blocking the ostium of the maxillary sinus.

A

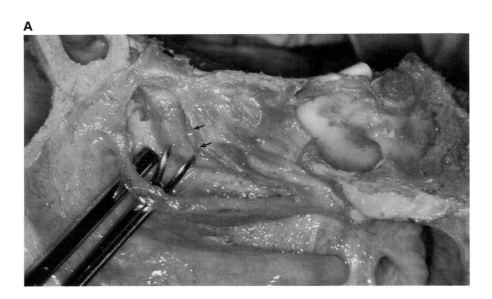

B

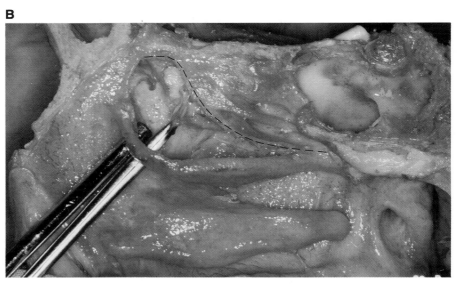

C

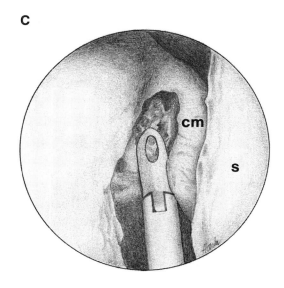

D

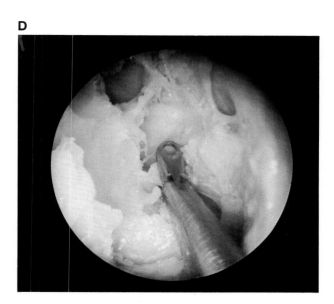

FIG 8–11.

A, anterior surface of the ethmoidal bulla is forced inward with a straight cup forceps. The *arrows* point to the cleft of the superior hiatus semilunaris and to the lateral sinus that is still hidden behind the remnants of the middle turbinate. For purposes of demonstration, the window in the middle turbinate had been enlarged. Note how far anteriorly and superiorly the path to the frontal recess and to the ostium of the frontal sinus goes. For the position of the endoscope selected for this preparation, the angle to the target is almost 90 degrees. *B,* bulla is opened and is being removed. The *dotted line* shows the course of the ground lamella of the middle turbinate. In this case it corresponds to the edge of the chosen window. **C,** drawing of the endoscopic view of the resection of the bulla. On first entering the bulla it is important to stay as far medially as possible. *cm* = middle turbinate, *s* = septum. **D,** removal of the smaller cellular septa and the remnants of the bulla from the ground lamella and the roof of the ethmoid. The roof of the ethmoid can be seen as a pale yellow structure directly above the forceps. At 11 o'clock, the passage through the frontal recess, in the direction of the frontal sinus, can be seen.

The bulla is opened by gently pushing in its anterior face in a medial direction with a delicate Blakesley-Weil forceps. If the lumen of the bulla is identified, the entire bulla can be resected step by step. Excessive force should never be used. The septa and the mucous membrane should never be torn or pulled out vigorously; instead, they should be removed gently with rotatory motion of the forceps. It is important to remove the medial wall of the bulla, which may be adherent to the middle turbinate or even hidden behind the "overhang" of the turbinate.

The ethmoidal bulla opening should always be opened as far medially as possible, and the resection should be continued only if a clear lumen can be identified or if some other disease process is found within the bulla. It is important to remember that the ethmoidal bulla is not always pneumatized. There may be only a bony ridge (called the torus lateralis by Grünwald and referred to in the Latin American literature as the promontorio). The bulla may also be small, or even absent. In these circumstances the trochlea of the orbit may be hidden behind a bulge in the lateral wall of the nose, and if this bulge is opened, the orbit is entered. This is usually not a serious complication, provided the bulging orbital fat is not mistaken for mucosa and removed.

Above and slightly anterior to the bulla there may be one to three usually distinct smaller ethmoidal cells. A larger space of variable size, the sinus lateralis (lateral sinus), may be present, extending between the bulla and the roof of the ethmoidal sinus medial to the lamina papyracea, lateral to the middle turbinate, and posteriorly between the bulla and the ground lamella of the middle turbinate (see Chapter 2).

If it is desirable to clean the roof of the ethmoidal sinus, the location of the anterior ethmoidal artery can usually be identified. This artery usually runs just below the roof of the ethmoidal sinus in a bony canal (which occasionally is dehiscent), across the anterior ethmoidal sinus on its way from the orbit to the olfactory fossa in the anterior base of the skull (for a more precise description of the anatomy of the anterior ethmoidal artery, see Chapter 2).

After the ethmoidal bulla and any of its adjacent cells have been removed (which is necessary only when these cells are diseased), the operative field is then bordered medially by the middle turbinate, laterally by the lamina papyracea, superiorly by the roof of the ethmoidal sinus, and posteriorly by the ground lamella of the middle turbinate.

If there is no sign of posterior ethmoidal disease but the frontal recess and the frontal sinus are diseased, their operative treatment is begun.

Perforation of Ground Lamella (Posterior Ethmoidectomy)

If the posterior ethmoidal sinus is also involved, it is now approached through the ground lamella of the middle turbinate. This ground lamella (basal lamella) divides the anterior ethmoidal sinus from the posterior ethmoidal sinus. Dehiscences and perforations of the ground lamella are the most common route through which disease spreads from the anterior to the posterior ethmoidal sinus.

After the ethmoidal bulla has been removed, the course of the ground lamella can usually be easily followed with the endoscope, commencing at the posterior end of the middle turbinate, where at the horizontal insertion of the middle turbinate it forms the roof of the middle meatus (Figs 8–12 and 8–13). Posterior to the ethmoidal bulla it curves superiorly into an almost vertical plane (approached sagittally by the endoscope) and inserts laterally into the lamina

A

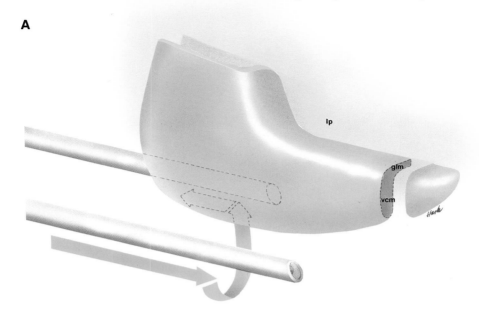

B

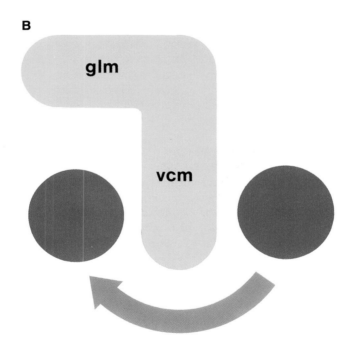

FIG 8–12.
A, schematic drawing of a right middle turbinate and its ground lamella. The insertion of the horizontal posterior portion, as well as of the middle frontal segment on the lamina papyracea, can be seen. The insertion of the anterior third is separated from the lamina papyracea and inserts vertically onto the base of the skull at the lateral edge of the lamina cribrosa, exactly across from its lateral lamella. A small segment has been excised from the posterior end of the middle turbinate to demonstrate the horizontal part of the ground lamella, which forms the roof of the middle meatus in its posterior aspect. *lp* = lamina papyracea; *glm* = ground lamella of the middle turbinate; *vcm* = the vertical portion of the middle turbinate. **B,** view of the resected edge of the middle turbinate showing the ground lamella and vertical portion of the middle turbinate relative to the positioning of the endoscope (end-on view). *glm* = ground lamella of the middle turbinate; *vcm* = vertical portion of the middle turbinate.

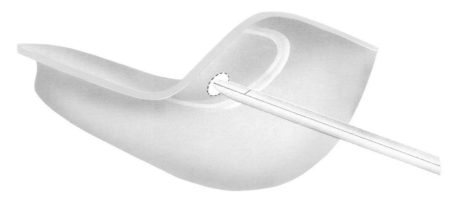

FIG 8–13.
Lateral schematic view of a middle turbinate and its ground lamella. The turbinate is shown here separate from the lamina papyracea. The ethmoidal bulla has already been removed (*ghosted white contour*). The ground lamella is being perforated with the straight cupped forceps 3 to 4 mm above the point at which it turns upward from its posterior horizontal course.

papyracea, and occasionally even onto the medial wall of the maxillary sinus. The ground lamella thus reaches the base of the skull. At this point its insertion extends medially for the last 1.5 to 2 cm and forms the vertical insertion of the middle turbinate at the base of the skull.

Identification of the ground lamella may be made difficult by pathologic changes or anatomic variations. If there is a prominent lateral sinus, it will extend between the posterior surface of the ethmoidal bulla and the ground lamella. If the lateral sinus is small or nonexistent, the posterior wall of the bulla frequently fuses to the ground lamella. In this case, perforation of the posterior wall of the ethmoidal bulla will open directly into the posterior ethmoidal sinus or into the superior meatus.

Identification of the ground lamella is made even more difficult because the lamella is not always a smooth, flat bony plate. Posterior ethmoidal cells may cause the lamella to bulge markedly anteriorly (i.e., into the lumen of the anterior ethmoidal sinus). Similarly, anterior ethmoidal cells, particularly when associated with an irregularly shaped lateral sinus, can dent the lamella in the direction of the posterior ethmoidal sinus. If such a cell is opened during the procedure on the anterior ethmoidal sinus, identification of the ground lamella and the beginning of the posterior ethmoidal sinus may be difficult.

If the posterior ethmoidal sinus must be opened, the ground lamella should be perforated as far medially and inferiorly as possible. The best place is 3 to 4 mm cranially from the point where the ground lamella turns superiorly from its horizontal course as the roof of the posterior third of the middle meatus just behind the ethmoidal bulla (see Fig 8–13). The ground lamella is carefully pushed inward, and the lumen behind it is identified before the opening is enlarged as needed (Fig 8–14). Under no circumstances should the entire ground lamella be removed, because this will destabilize the middle turbinate.

The posterior ethmoidal sinus is now freely accessible, and the surgeon can determine if the mucosa need to be resected. When working in the posterior ethmoidal sinus, the surgeon must always keep in mind that a markedly pneumatized posterior ethmoidal sinus may lie in intimate contact with the optic nerve laterally. The lamina papyracea, as the lateral border of the posterior ethmoidal sinus, extends posteriorly as a triangular plate that corresponds to the apex of the orbit. In a surprisingly large number of patients, the extension

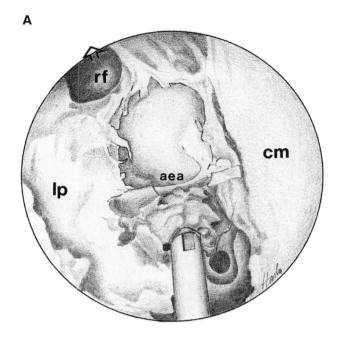

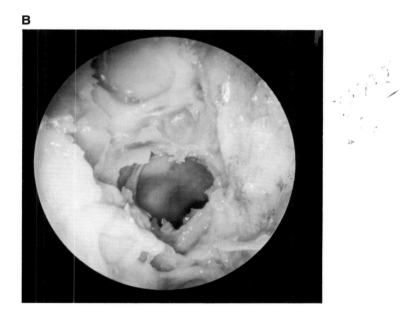

FIG 8–14.
A, appearance after perforation of the ground lamella. After the perforation is made to identify the posterior ethmoidal sinus (the round opening at 5 o'clock on the right below and alongside the forceps), additional portions of the ground lamella are removed. *rf* = frontal recess; *lp* = lamina papyracea; *aea* = anterior ethmoidal artery; *cm* = middle turbinate. **B,** endoscopic picture showing the appearance after the hole in the ground lamella has been enlarged. There is now an unobstructed view into the posterior ethmoidal sinus, and the roof of the ethmoid can be clearly identified. The dangers of inadvertent injury are largely eliminated once the roof of the ethmoid has been clearly identified anterior and posterior to the anterior ethmoidal artery, and the artery itself has also been identified. If indicated, it is now possible to remove additional cellular septa and disease in the immediate vicinity of the ethmoidal artery at the skull base.

of the tip of this triangle posteriorly shows a bulge in the posterior ethmoidal sinus under which the optic nerve runs.

The angle of the endoscope must change as the surgeon proceeds deeper into the ethmoidal sinus (Fig 8–15). The 0-degree endoscope should have been at a 45-degree angle to the palate when the infundibulum was opened. Now, just before the anterior wall of the ground lamella, the endoscope should lie at a 30-degree angle to the palate. This change in angulation of the endoscope allows the surgeon to follow the path along the base of the skull.

Tips for Identification of Correct Point for Perforation of Ground Lamella

When the ground lamella must be perforated to gain access to the posterior ethmoidal sinus, the safest place to do so can be found in the following way.

After the ethmoidal bulla has been resected, the posterior third of the middle meatus is identified through the endoscope. Its roof here is formed by the almost horizontally running ground lamella. This roof is followed from posterior to anterior, and the point at which the ground lamella changes orientation from horizontal to almost vertical, and at which point it bends sharply superiorly behind the (previously removed) ethmoidal bulla, is identified. Three to 4 mm superior from this turn, the perforation is made, as far medial as possible, to reach the superior meatus and the posterior ethmoidal sinus. In this way, the danger of getting too close to or even perforating the roof of the ethmoidal sinus can be avoided. This danger is particularly great when there is a lateral sinus that extends far posteriorly or that invaginates the ground lamella posteriorly and superiorly.

This perforation is created by pushing the instrument, usually a small Blakesley forceps, through the bony lamella, with the jaws closed. Once through the lamella, the jaws are opened and the opening is identified and then enlarged. The lumen must always be clearly identified before a cutting or biting instrument is used.

A

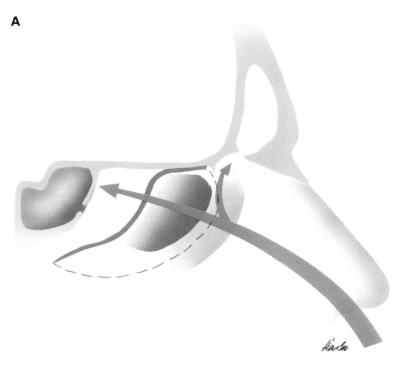

B

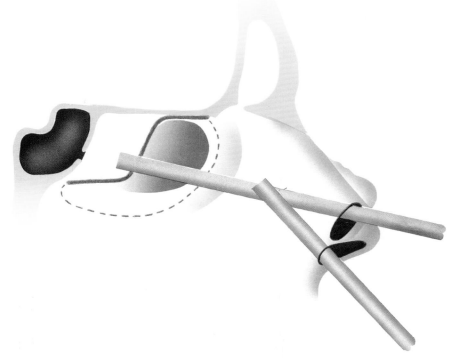

FIG 8–15.
A, schematic drawing of the endoscopic procedure. The path of the instruments is shown as a *gray arrow* assuming that an advance to the sphenoid sinus is necessary or that the frontal recess needs to be entered for some manipulation anterior to the bulla and in an anterosuperior direction. **B,** schematic drawing illustrating the change in angulation of the endoscope required as it advances into the ethmoidal sinus. Initially, the endoscope is introduced at an angle of about 45 degrees to the hard palate, this angle deceases as the instrument is advanced posteriorly. Depending on the anatomic conditions, the final angle of the endoscope at the anterior wall of the sphenoid sinus is in the range of 15 to 25 degrees to the hard palate.

Sphenoidectomy

If the sphenoidal sinus must be opened, the surgeon should remember that the path through the ethmoidal sinus does not lead to the anterior wall of the sphenoidal sinus in the region of its natural ostium, but further superiorly and laterally. In cases of isolated involvement of this sinus, its natural ostium can be approached through the sphenoethmoidal recess, medial to the turbinates, via the nasal cavity. In some cases of pneumatization the cells of the posterior ethmoidal sinus may extend far laterally from the sphenoidal sinus, and may even extend over it as Onodi cells (see Chapters 2 and 11). Onodi cells are usually pyramidal, with the base of the pyramid facing anteriorly (toward the surgeon). Under no circumstances should the anterior wall of the sphenoidal sinus be sought behind such a lateral extrusion of the posterior ethmoidal sinus, because of the close proximity to the optic nerve.

When the anterior wall of the sphenoidal sinus must be opened, this must be done as far medially and inferiorly as possible. The anterior wall of the sphenoidal sinus can be indented with a delicate bent spoon, the lumen of the sphenoid sinus identified, and finally, as much of the anterior wall removed as is required for the proposed procedure and which can be safely accomplished (Fig 8–16).

In any operation on the posterior ethmoidal or sphenoidal sinus, it is particularly important for the surgeon to study the tomograms preoperatively and to become thoroughly familiar with the relationships between the optic nerve, the internal carotid artery, and the sphenoidal sinus. The greatest care must be taken when working near the lateral wall and the roof of the sphenoidal sinus. In any attempt to perforate or remove septa in the sphenoidal sinus, the surgeon must be certain that these septa are not adjacent and do not insert onto the canal of the internal carotid artery or the optic nerve.

A

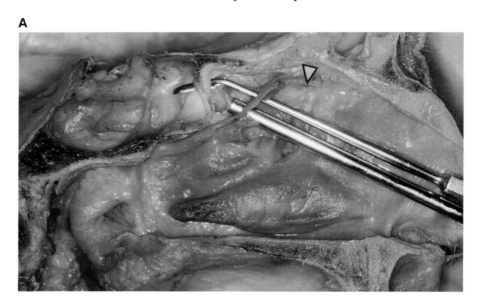

B

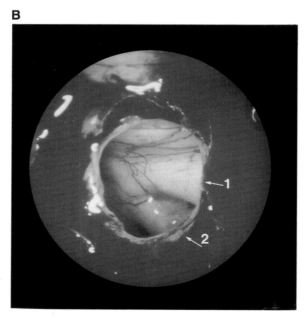

C

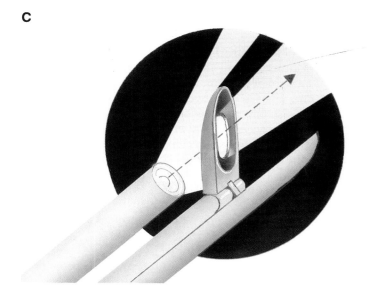

D

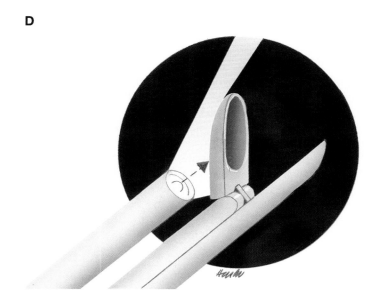

FIG 8–16.
A, tip of the 0-degree endoscope has passed through the ground lamella of the middle turbinate (resected here for demonstration purposes) and is located in the posterior ethmoidal sinus. The anterior surface of the sphenoid sinus is carefully depressed with a bent spoon. Note the position of the spoon, with the bend *downward.* The *triangular arrow* indicates the position of the anterior ethmoidal artery. **B,** endoscopic view with a zero-degree endoscope through an operatively opened left sphenoid sinus. The course of the optic nerve, coming from the apex of the orbit and underneath the somewhat posterior course of the internal carotid artery, can be seen clearly. 1 = optic nerve; 2 = internal carotid artery. **C,** in these delicate maneuvers, minor details may become important. Thus, for instance, the window in the jaws of the Blakesley-Weil forceps may permit a view through the jaws of the forceps if the endoscope is brought close to the fenestration. **D,** this is not possible in the otherwise similar Takahashi forceps.

If the sphenoidal sinus is only minimally diseased or is not diseased, the bulge of the optic nerve canal usually can be seen on the lateral wall just below the roof. (Occasionally the bulge of the optic nerve may be seen in the posterior ethmoidal sinus.) Below the optic nerve the more or less prominent bulge of the internal carotid artery can be seen in its course in the cavernous sinus (see Fig 8–16). The distance between the carotid artery and the optic nerve is determined by the degree of pneumatization of the sphenoidal sinus. The surgeon must always remember that in 25% of patients the bone over the carotid artery is clinically dehiscent. This means that in histologic sections a paper-thin layer of bone may be found over the artery, but as far as the palpating instrument is concerned, the vessel is covered only with periosteum and mucous membrane. Under no circumstances in this area, and especially in revision procedures where scars may cover the area, should cutting instruments, curettes, or punch forceps be used carelessly.

Tips for Identification of Sphenoidal Sinus

After passing through the anterior and posterior ethmoidal sinuses, the anterior wall of the sphenoid sinus is always encountered much more medially and inferiorly than originally anticipated. To enter the anterior wall of the sphenoidal sinus, the same technique is used as described for the ground lamella. A small, angled spoon is suitable for this purpose, although it should always be used with its angled end pointing downward (see Fig 8–16).

Even with minimal pneumatization, the most posterior ethmoidal air cells will lie lateral to the sphenoidal sinus, and as a result, the anterior wall of the sphenoidal sinus is no longer in a frontal plane but runs at an acute angle from anteromedial to posterolateral. If the anterior wall of the sphenoidal sinus cannot be definitely identified, it is usually possible to find its natural ostium, medial to all of the turbinates, through the sphenoethmoidal recess and to enlarge the sphenoidal sinus ostium inferiorly. This procedure requires the placement of anesthetic pledgets into the sphenoethmoidal recess. We use this approach in those cases of isolated sphenoidal sinus disease that require surgical management.

We do not in the framework of the Messerklinger technique perform direct diagnostic sphenoidal sinus endoscopy through a modified maxillary sinus trocar, as described by Draf. When it is necessary to take a biopsy specimen from the sphenoidal sinus, we use the technique described earlier, that is, across the sphenoethmoidal recess, through the enlarged sphenoidal sinus ostium under direct endoscopic vision.

Opening Frontal Recess

For opening the frontal recess, we use a delicate angled Blakesley-Weil forceps and the 30-degree nasal endoscope (Fig 8–17). The angled forceps can usually be advanced superiorly, below the insertion of the middle turbinate, and the involved mucous membrane and cellular septa removed. The exact technique depends in each case on the highly variable anatomic configuration of this area (see Chapter 2). It is usually possible to gain a good look into the frontal sinus without having to manipulate the ostium itself after the cranial extensions of the uncinate process have been removed.

In cases of extensive pneumatization and involvement of the agger nasi or when the uncinate process bends laterally and inserts onto the lamina papyracea (with the formation of a terminal recess of the infundibulum), localization of the ostium of the frontal sinus may be very difficult. In the first case, the incision to resect the uncinate process can be carried further superiorly, beyond the insertion of the middle turbinate (Fig 8–18). From here it is possible to clean the agger nasi cells and obtain a better view of the anatomy of the frontal recess. If the uncinate process and the agger nasi extend far medially, the path to the ostium of the frontal sinus may be a very narrow slit, located medially between the uncinate process and the middle turbinate.

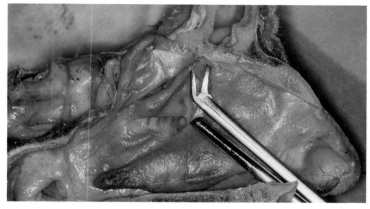

FIG 8–17.
For work in the frontal recess we prefer to use a 30-degree lens and a variety of curved Blakesley-Weil forceps. This illustration shows how the frontal recess may be treated without requiring resection of the ethmoidal bulla. For purposes of demonstration, the middle turbinate is deflected upward. A superior remnant of the uncinate process is being removed with the upbiting forceps.

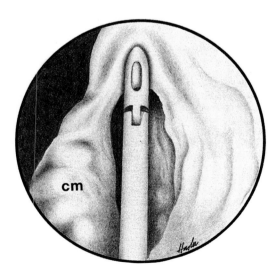

FIG 8–18.
If the agger nasi is pneumatized, it may become necessary to open it or, as in this illustration, to dissect it along the insertion of the middle turbinate to reach the frontal recess more easily. This may result in oozing from the terminal branches of the ethmoidal artery that run inferiorly in the mucosa of this region. For this reason we try to avoid this procedure. *cm* = middle turbinate.

A

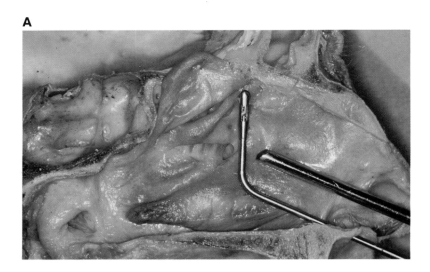

B

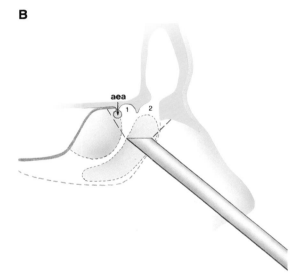

FIG 8–19.
A, variety of upturned forceps, which are available with a variety of angles and with both horizontal and vertical jaws, are also suitable for this purpose. **B,** once the anterior ethmoidal artery has been identified, the 30-degree lens usually shows a small recess that is present directly in front of the artery. This recess is easily mistaken for the route to the frontal sinus, particularly if it widens into a supraorbital recess. Typically the actual route to the frontal sinus is farther anterior, separated from this recess by a bony ridge. *aea* = anterior ethmoidal artery; *1* = a small recess directly anterior to the anterior ethmoidal artery; *2* = the actual route to the frontal sinus.

Depending on the degree of pneumatization of the frontal sinus, the axis through the ostium of the frontal sinus and the frontal recess may be angled fairly far forward. This means that the path for the surgeon is first posterosuperiorly under the insertion of the middle turbinate, then anterosuperiorly to the ostium of the frontal sinus (Fig 8–19). When conditions are very restricted and the ethmoidal infundibulum ends in a terminal recess, work in this area may be the most difficult part of the entire procedure. In these cases the frequently slitlike entrance to the frontal recess lies much more medial (i.e., closer to the middle turbinate than expected). When working in this area, the surgeon must always remember that one is close to the thinnest and most fragile portion of the anterior base of the skull: the medial precipice of the ethmoid in the area of the exit of the anterior ethmoidal artery.

If it is difficult to identify the ostium of the frontal sinus, yet the pathologic findings require that this be done, the surgeon should always try to visualize the anterior ethmoidal artery and then to dissect forward from this area in a retrograde fashion. In front of the anterior ethmoidal artery there is usually a small extension of the ethmoid roof that can open into a supraorbital recess (see Fig 8–19). If deep, this recess may be mistaken for the frontal sinus. As a rule, the sinus is usually anterior to the recess (see Chapter 2). Under no circumstances should any pressure be exerted superiorly or medially with any instrument introduced into the frontal recess.

Occasionally it is impossible to place both the endoscope and the instrument under the medial turbinate simultaneously and thus be able to view and work simultaneously. In such cases, the surgeon may try to remove a part of the insertion of the middle turbinate from the lateral wall of the nose with an angled Blakesley forceps. The disadvantage of this maneuver may be slight hemorrhage that further impedes the view. With experience it becomes possible to look into the frontal recess with the angled lens, identify the part to be removed, then withdraw the endoscope a few millimeters to make room for the introduction of the instrument. After removal of the tissue or bony segment, the endoscope is again advanced and the recess reinspected. This procedure requires the greatest caution, and may be the most demanding for the surgeon.

Occasionally the path to the frontal sinus is indicated by the presence of abnormal secretions. Tiny bubbles appearing in the blood droplets during surgery on the frontal recess may also be of assistance.

A good view of the inside of the frontal sinus can now be gained with the 30- or 70-degree endoscope (see Fig 8–17). In cases of isolated cysts or polyps, the sinus can be entered through the ostium, and the growth removed through the ostium. Disease located laterally within the frontal sinus usually cannot be approached via this route.

We do not routinely enlarge the ostium of the frontal sinus. In patients with an isolated frontal recess problem, the last surgical steps can be performed after the uncinate process has been resected and without touching the ethmoidal bulla or any of the other deeper structures.

Tips for Identification of Frontal Recess

When difficulties are encountered in visualizing the ostium of the frontal sinus "around the corner" anterosuperiorly from below the insertion of the middle turbinate, it is helpful to ask the patient to extend the head (i.e., to raise the chin). This small change in position frequently improves visibility in the frontal recess markedly. When working in the frontal recess, we prefer the Blakesley-Weil instruments. Their fenestrated jaws allow a view of the structures behind them. This is particularly helpful when the tip of the endoscope must be very close to the jaws of the instrument.

When we are unable to identify the ostium of the frontal sinus because of extensive scarring from previous operations or because the landmarks, such as the middle turbinate, have been removed, it is possible to perform a Beck procedure (frontal trephination) and thus to view the floor of the frontal sinus. At the same time, an angled Blakesley forceps can be introduced into the frontal recess intranasally. When the tip of this instrument produces a bulge in the floor of the sinus, this point can usually be safely used to perforate the scar tissue plate. Normally the periphery of the frontal sinus is manipulated as little as possible with the Messerklinger technique. Therefore, massive scar tissue, bony obstruction, or stenoses of the ostium of the frontal sinus are not indications for use of the Messerklinger technique.

If the frontal recess is involved by massive polyposis and there are no anatomic landmarks, it is sometimes helpful to introduce anesthetic and decongestant pledgets repeatedly after the polypectomy. After a few minutes, endoscopic examination may identify small trickles of secretions and thus lead the surgeon directly to the ostium of the frontal sinus.

The cone of light projected by the 30-degree lens may also be useful in pointing the way to the frontal sinus. Holding the endoscope in the chosen position and inspecting the area of the frontal sinus from the outside, the surgeon often can see that the light transilluminates the frontal sinus, even though the endonasal route has not yet been clearly identified. The 30-degree angle between the shaft of the endoscope and the direction of the light beam may then provide a guide in identifying the proper route to the frontal sinus ostium.

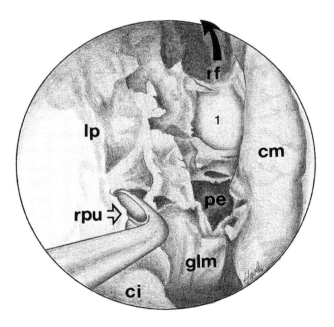

FIG 8–20.
To locate the ostium of the maxillary sinus, we first identify the remnants of the uncinate process with a bent spoon. The ostium is usually found laterally and below, between these remnants and the almost always identifiable insertion of the bulla lamella. The safest technique is to stay so far inferiorly as to ride on the bony insertion of the inferior turbinate. *cm* = middle turbinate; *lp* = lamina papyracea; *rf* = frontal recess with path to the frontal sinus (*arrow*); *pe* = view into the posterior ethmoidal sinus through a perforation in the ground lamella; *rpu* = remnants of the uncinate process; *glm* = horizontal portion of the ground lamella serving as a roof to the posterior third of the middle meatus; *ci* = inferior turbinate; *1* = "dome" of the roof of the ethmoid.

Identification of Natural Ostium of Maxillary Sinus

If the disease process requires it, the next step is localization and enlargement of the natural ostium of the maxillary sinus. If the ostium has not yet become visible, it is either closed or covered by diseased mucous membrane or is hidden by a posteroinferior remnant of the uncinate process (Fig. 8–20). The best way to find the ostium of the maxillary sinus is by careful palpation with a bent spoon along the bony insertion of the inferior turbinate. This leads either into the ostium itself or into one of the fontanelles. The surgeon should never palpate too far superiorly (to prevent breaching into the orbit through the lamina papyracea). Frequently, small bubbles emerging from between folds of mucosa, from between polyps, or from a pool of blood will reveal the site of the ostium.

Once identified, the ostium can be enlarged with a bent spoon, a small curette, or a pair of backbiting forceps. The appropriate instrument is introduced into the ostium and pulled anteroinferiorly, in the direction of the anterior fontanelle (at whose expense the natural ostium is enlarged). In the area of the fontanelle there is no bone between the mucosa of the maxillary sinus and that of the middle meatus, and thus enlargement of the ostium can be accomplished with ease. The ostium can be trimmed to the desired shape with a reverse cutting (backbiting) punch forceps. If accessory ostia are present in one of the fontanelles, the accessory ostium and the natural ostium should be united to prevent the circular transportation of secretions (described in Chapter 1). Anteriorly the bony nasolacrimal duct limits the enlargement of the ostium. This bone is considerably harder than any other in this area and thus is easy to identify. It must be remembered, however, that the reverse cutting punch forceps is a strong instrument and can remove even this hard bone.

With the appropriate instruments (angled suction tips or special malleable forceps), under the guidance of a 30- or 70-degree nasal endoscope, some procedures can be performed inside the maxillary sinus through its natural or enlarged ostium (Fig 8–21). These procedures may include removal of an isolated large symptomatic cyst or pedunculated polyp or evacuation of retained secretions. We usually do not touch extensive polypoid changes. Figure 8–21 shows the position of the enlarged natural ostium in the middle meatus and the excellent view that it permits into the maxillary sinus. The course of the infraorbital nerve is clearly visible. Enlargement of the natural ostium of the maxillary sinus is not a routine component of endoscopic ethmoidal surgery, and is carried out only when required by pathologic and anatomic conditions.

Work in the maxillary sinus can be undertaken from two sides using a bimeatal procedure. The trocar sheath left in the maxillary sinus after preliminary endoscopic exploration through the canine fossa can now be used to removal single polyps from the wall of the sinus. The polyp is manipulated by the trocar sheath toward the ostium, where it can be grasped with the suction tip or angled forceps and removed. We use this approach most commonly for removal of mycotic masses from the maxillary sinus.

Tips for Identification of Ostium of Maxillary Sinus

If the natural ostium of the maxillary sinus cannot be seen after resection of the uncinate process, this is probably because of edematous mucous membrane or, more commonly, posteroinferior remnants of the uncinate process. These uncinate remnants should be identified and removed.

Pressure against the fontanelles may make bubbles appear through the natural ostium and thereby reveal its location. When locating the ostium of the

A

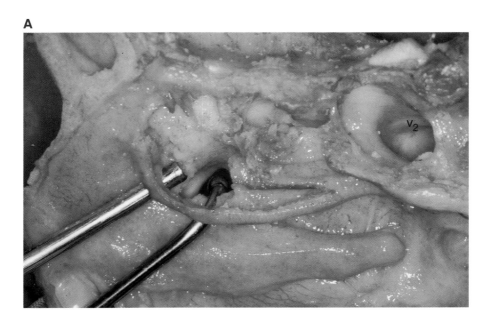

B

C

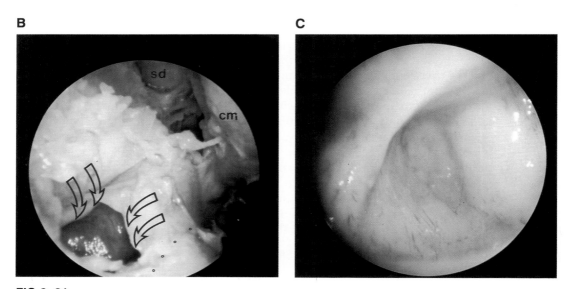

FIG 8–21.
A, view of a surgically enlarged maxillary sinus ostium through which procedures can be performed inside the sinus V_2 = groove of the second branch of the trigeminal nerve in the lateral wall of the sphenoid sinus. **B,** appearance after enlargement of the natural ostium of the maxillary sinus (*arrows*). The *dotted line* corresponds to the line of insertion of the inferior turbinate. **C,** view into the maxillary sinus through the natural ostium with a 70-degree lens. The course of the infraorbital nerve can be seen clearly, curving inferiorly from the roof of the maxillary sinus to the infraorbital foramen on the anterior wall of the sinus.

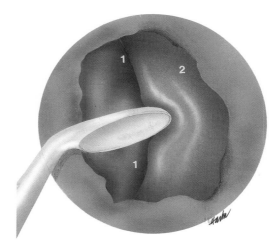

FIG 8–22.
The situation after an alleged opening of the ostium of a left maxillary sinus. The medial bony wall of the maxillary sinus is fenestrated, and the surgeon assumes that he or she is looking into the lumen of the maxillary sinus (*1*). In fact, the spoon is elevating the mucosa (*2*) of the maxillary sinus laterally and anteriorly in toto and thus denuding the posterior wall and, occasionally, even the roof of the maxillary sinus (*1*). In reality then, one is looking into a space between the maxillary sinus mucosa and the posterior wall of the maxillary sinus.

maxillary sinus, it is best to palpate along the bony insertion of the inferior turbinate into the lateral nasal wall. This prevents accidental perforation of the orbit.

Similarly to the frontal sinus, it is possible to locate and enlarge the natural ostium from the inner side of the lumen through the maxillary sinus. By maxillary sinus endoscopy through the canine fossa, the ostium can be inspected while a bent spoon is used to palpate from the middle meatus. This further minimizes the danger of creating a perforation in the wrong place.

Occasionally the maxillary sinus mucosa may be elevated and pushed laterally from the medial wall or elevated from the roof of the sinus by the palpating spoon or other instrument. This situation is difficult to recognize. The lumen that becomes visible actually corresponds to the space between the displaced mucosa and the bone, when in fact the sinus has not yet been entered (Fig 8–22). Once this mistake has been recognized, it is frequently difficult to grasp the displaced mucosa, because attempts usually just displace it further laterally. In this event, opening of the sinus is best accomplished with an angled Blakesley suction forceps, with which the mucosa can both be held (suction) and opened. Only now should the newly created window be enlarged.

Another option is to close the nostril with gentle pressure over the endoscope and the instrument and ask the patient to inhale. The negative pressure created by inhalation may cause the mucosa to bulge medially, making it easier to grasp.

Summary

Total sphenoethmoidectomy can be performed by the Messerklinger technique without resection of the middle turbinate (Fig 8–23). We rarely perform total sphenoethmoidectomy, but when we do, we see no need to remove the entire mucous membrane. We take great care, however, to assure that the connections between the compartments are patent. With the Messerklinger technique, it is not necessary to perform "cosmetic" surgery; in other words, there is no need to smooth and polish the roof of the ethmoid with a diamond drill or to totally

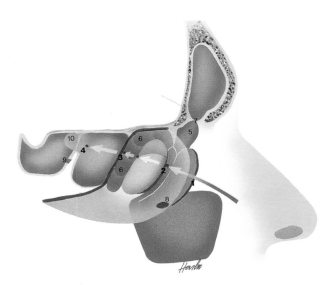

FIG 8–23.
Schematic drawing illustrating the four primary lamellae that must be crossed in an almost frontal plane on the way to the sphenoid sinus: *1* = uncinate process; *2* = anterior wall of the ethmoidal bulla (*pink*); *3* = ground lamella of the middle turbinate; and *4* = anterior wall of the sphenoidal sinus. Between *3* and *4*, an additional ground lamella of the superior (and occasionally of the supreme) turbinate may be encountered. These structures are not always present and do not have the clinical significance of the ground lamella of the middle turbinate. *5* = frontal recess; *6* = lateral sinus; *7* = ostium of the frontal sinus; *8* = ostium of the maxillary sinus; *9* = ostium of the sphenoidal sinus. The frontal recess (*5*) and the lateral sinus (*6*) are only incompletely separated in this case by a vertical bony ridge. *10* = the projection of the posterior ethmoidal cell onto the lateral wall of the sphenoidal sinus (described by Onodi). The outline of the middle turbinate is indicated by *gray ghosting*.

remove all of the cellular septa. This will only create uncovered bony surfaces, which in turn cause delayed healing, with granulation tissue, occasionally marked crust formation, or even osteitis. Such action may also endanger the ethmoidal vessels, requiring the use of packs, which in themselves will increase mucosal injury and lead to synechia formation. Care must be taken, however, that no recesses or spaces remain that could close off and become the site of renewed retention or a fresh nidus for disease.

PREVENTING INJURY TO ORBITS

Surgeons who perform endonasal procedures with the patient under general anesthesia emphasize the need for the patient's eyes be visible to the surgeon or the scrub nurse at all times. This may make it possible to recognize injury to the orbit by movement of the eyeball or by the appearance of an intraorbital hematoma.

In most cases, encroachment of the orbit can be recognized by the identification of orbital fat, which can be distinguished from diseased mucosa by the fat's yellow color (Fig 8–24). A less direct sign may be the presence of small fatty "eyes" (readily recognized through the endoscope) on the blood droplets in the ethmoidal sinus.

Even prolapse of orbital fat usually does not cause significant complications. If the periorbital tissues are only split, an attempt may be made to replace the fat very carefully with a blunt instrument. *Under no circumstances should the fat be pulled out or resected.* At the end of the procedure, the prolapsed fat can be "splinted" with a small Merocel sponge, kept in place for 1 to 3 days. The patient should be instructed not to blow the nose (to avoid orbital emphysema), and antibiotics are prescribed.

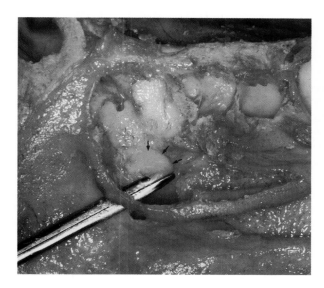

FIG 8–24.
Perforation of the orbit and protrusion of orbital fat (*arrows*). The lesion in the lamina papyracea is located in the characteristic site. The orbit can be injured in this area when the sickle knife is carried too far laterally against the lamina papyracea during resection of the uncinate process.

Injury to the orbit occurs most commonly at the time of the initial incision to open the infundibulum (resection of the uncinate process), on removing the ethmoidal bulla, and during the search for and enlargement of the ostium of the maxillary sinus. Pain is an important warning sign. Injury to the periorbital area will be felt by the patient as pain in the eye. This warning sign is absent when general anesthesia is used.

All tissue removed from the nose during the procedure should be placed by the nurse into a small container filled with normal saline or Ringer's solution. The nurse should be instructed to advise the surgeon immediately if any of the tissue floats in the solution. Such tissue should be immediately inspected. It could be a small portion of mucous membrane with a small air bubble caught in it. Pushing the tissue a few times with an instrument and turning it over should release the air, and the tissue should then sink to the bottom. The only tissue that may float naturally is fat and brain.

PAIN

It surprises us how little local anesthetic is required to reach the sphenoidal sinus, even when the injections are limited to the mucous membrane of the uncinate process and to the insertion of the middle turbinate. In addition to the use of an appropriate analgesic and sedative premedication, the most important factors in providing freedom from pain are correct application and adequate contact time of the anesthetic pledgets. There are some points, however, where even a well-anesthetized patient will feel pain. These include the roof of the ethmoid, particularly in the area of the ethmoidal vessels and nerves, the medial wall of the orbit, the area around the ostium of the maxillary sinus, and especially the posterior end of the middle turbinate.

The area of the anterior ethmoidal nerve is highly sensitive. This nerve occasionally accompanies the artery, either anteriorly or posteriorly, and may divide into two or more branches. If the patient who was previously free of pain complains of pain after the ethmoidal bulla has been removed, the surgeon should make sure about the anatomic relationships. The ethmoid roof is significantly more sensitive to pain than any of the adjacent areas.

When a patient who is uncomfortable throughout the entire procedure is asked where it hurts, the answer is frequently "Just where you are working"; in other words, there is diffuse localization. If, however, the periorbital area is touched or injured, the response will be immediate: "I feel pain in the eye." Pain provides the most important warning sign, and helps to prevent the more serious complications. This advantage is lost when general anesthesia is used.

The area around the natural ostium of the maxillary sinus, particularly its inferior and posterior margins, can be very pain sensitive. This can be remedied by injecting anesthetic below the mucosa of the most posterior extensions of the uncinate process. Anesthetic can also be injected into the mucosa over the posterior fontanelle when topical anesthesia is not sufficient.

The posterior end of the middle turbinate can also be very pain sensitive. Frequently only 2 to 3 mm above this area the vessels and nerves from the sphenopalatine foramen emerge and advance into the mucosa of the turbinates and into the lateral wall of the nose. One of the few situations in which the Messerklinger technique is used in this area is for opening and resection of a concha bullosa, when the pneumatization of the middle turbinate extends to the posterior end of the middle turbinate, or if the lateral lamella of the concha bullosa has to be resected as far as this point. There is danger of direct injury to the vessels and nerves in this area. The additional injection of local anesthetic may be helpful even after the concha has already been opened. Removal of the most posterior fragments of the lateral lamella of the turbinate is better tolerated when performed by sharp dissection (scissors or a modified conchotome) rather than by pulling, tugging, and twisting with a Blakesley forceps.

The application of local anesthesia may be particularly difficult in those patients who have undergone previous surgery for diffuse, polypoid rhinosinopathy with extensive scar formation from which new polyps originate. The best solution in these patients is to repeatedly apply the anesthetic and vasoconstrictor pledgets and to operate in a ping-pong fashion. The anesthetic pledgets are placed in one side while the surgeon operates on the other side, and vice versa. In repeat operations, it is helpful to inject the scarred stalk of the new polyps with a small amount of local anesthetic and then resect them with sharp dissection.

Another source of pain may be introduction of the suction tip into an ethmoidal cell or into a sinus through a small opening that fits tightly around the suctioner. When suction is applied, the sudden negative pressure in the closed space may produce sudden sharp pain. It is therefore important to ensure that air can enter the space around the suction tip, to prevent creation of an area of negative pressure.

ENDOSCOPIC RESECTION OF CONCHA BULLOSA

If a concha bullosa contributes to ethmoidal disease or is itself diseased, the first step is resection of its lateral half. The medial lamella, which serves as the attachment of the turbinate to the roof of the ethmoidal sinus and, via the ground lamella, to the lamina papyracea, is left alone to create the most physiologic conditions possible. Depending on the extent of pneumatization of the middle turbinate, it may be necessary to extend the procedure as far as the posterior end of the turbinate.

If it is not certain that the lateral nasal wall will also require surgical intervention (e.g., resection of the uncinate process and removal of the ethmoidal bulla), only the mucosa over the concha bullosa should be infiltrated with local anesthetic. This prevents oozing from the puncture sites over the uncinate process and allows for better evaluation of the anterior ethmoidal clefts after removal of the lateral lamella of the concha bullosa.

Local anesthetic is administered at three to four sites in the insertion, on the anterior surface, and along the free inferior margin of the turbinate. If the mucosa is thin and the bony plate of the turbinate is also thin, the needle may break through into a turbinate cell. Great care must be taken that the local anesthetic is deposited between the mucous membrane and the bony surface of the concha bullosa.

The turbinate air cell is then entered with a curved blade in the area of the most pronounced pneumatization (Fig 8–25). This area may be located fairly far posterior in some cases. It is usually obvious when the tip of the blade drops into the turbinate cell. The incision is then carried downward along the free inferior margin with a sawing motion. After this, the cutting edge of the blade is turned superiorly and the incision extended to the insertion of the middle turbinate. If the insertion of the middle turbinate is delicate, great care should be taken not to break off the turbinate during these perforation maneuvers. This is particularly likely when the bony shell of the turbinate cell is very hard. In these cases, it is advisable to open the turbinate cell with straight scissors or a Struyken conchotome; this prevents direct pressure on the insertion of the turbinate. In displacement of the lateral lamella of the concha superiorly, care must be taken to keep the upper jaw of the scissors lateral to the insertion of the turbinate. The two leaves of the turbinate can usually be easily spread with the scissors, and a good view can be gained into the interior of the turbinate cell, revealing any mucosal pathologic conditions that may be present. Frequently the cell of a concha bullosa can be entered with the endoscope, and the ostium of the cell (i.e., point of origin of its pneumatization) can be identified.

The lateral lamella of the concha bullosa can then be grasped with a delicate, straight Blakesly forceps, sheared off with a careful rotatory, maneuver and

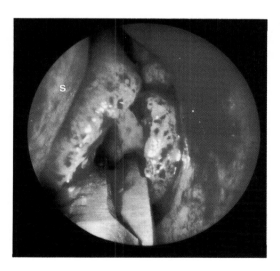

FIG 8–25.
The incision is carried along the inferior margin with scissors.

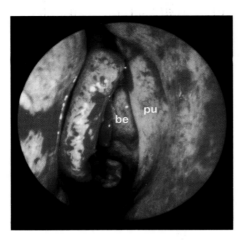

FIG 8–26.
After removal of most of the lateral lamella, a good view of the middle meatus can be obtained. *be* = ethmoidal bulla; *pu* = uncinate process.

removed. Total removal is not always possible if the middle turbinate is extensively pneumatized. In such cases, the lateral lamella must be removed piece by piece with the scissors and the straight Blakesly forceps. The closer the posterior end of the middle turbinate, the greater the risk of hemorrhage and pain, because the sphenopalatine foramen with its vessels and nerves is adjacent to this area.

After removal of most of the lateral lamella of the concha bullosa, a good view of the middle meatus is possible (Fig 8–26). Depending on the pathologic condition present, the procedure may be limited to the resection of the lateral lamella of the concha bullosa. The advantage of an endoscopic procedure is that intraoperative staging is always possible. The surgeon can decide on the spot whether the edematous mucosa is in the hiatus semilunaris or over the bulla and whether the infundibulum is narrow and requires additional surgical intervention. Should this be the case, an additional 1 mL of local anesthetic solution should be injected under the mucosa of the uncinate process before continuing the operation. Before proceeding, one must ascertain that the lateral lamella of the concha bullosa has been removed completely and that only the medial half remains.

If in addition to the resection of a concha bullosa the lateral nasal wall must also be treated, opposing wound surfaces will automatically be created. If the middle meatus is constricted or there has been unintentional injury to the head of the middle turbinate, we recommend that a small Merocel sponge moistened with beclomethasone be placed in the middle meatus for 1 or 2 days to prevent adhesions. Such cases must be monitored and followed closely to recognize the formation of adhesions and to treat them in a timely fashion. These adhesions may appear only after a few weeks, and they always extend from the insertion of the middle turbinate inferiorly.

9 Postoperative Care

We do not routinely insert packing into the middle meatus or the nose at the conclusion of the surgical procedure, because there is usually little, if any, bleeding. At the end of the procedure, the surgical area is examined with the endoscope and the larger clots removed. If an area of capillary oozing is identified (which occurs most commonly when the surgery was performed because of acute or chronic inflammation), we place a small piece of Oxycel absorbable mesh (100% regenerated oxidized cellulose; Johnson & Johnson) over the bleeding site. The Oxycel mesh can easily be draped over the bleeding surface, where it will immediately adhere to the raw surface and in most instances control the bleeding. Care should be taken that the ostia are not blocked by the mesh. The Oxycel mesh is usually absorbed within a few days.

Finally, the nasopharynx is carefully inspected, and any clots that may have accumulated in this area are removed with the aspirator. We routinely place a cotton pledget into the nasal vestibules to prevent blood-tinged secretions from running down the patient's face during the first few postoperative hours. The patient is instructed to remove the cotton after a few hours.

In those cases where opposing wound surfaces are created or where the middle meatus is extremely narrow, we usually place strips of compressed Merocel sponge into the middle meatus, which are then expanded by moistening them with a beclomethasone solution (e.g., Beconase aqueous solution). The strips of Merocel sponge are transfixed with a suture, and the end of the suture is taped to the patient's cheek. These sponges are kept in place for no more than 1 or 2 days, and during this time they must be kept moist with repeated application of beclomethasone solution several times each day.

It is important to inform the patient that the presence of some blood-tinged secretions in the nasopharynx is perfectly normal during the first few postoperative hours. These secretions should be gently expectorated, not swallowed. This makes it easier for the recovery room nurse to monitor blood loss and to recognize any fresh bleeding.

The patient is also requested not to blow the nose at all during the first 48 hours after surgery. This instruction must be emphasized and strictly followed by the patient, especially if maxillary sinus endoscopy was performed through the canine fossa or if the lamina papyracea has been breached during the procedure. If the patient needs to clear the nasal passages, sniffing inwardly as frequently as necessary is recommended.

During the first few days, physical exertion (e.g., lifting heavy objects) and all activities that could elevate blood pressure and thus increase perfusion of the surgical site must be avoided. The patient should be informed that after the topical and local anesthesia wears off, there should be little pain. For the first few hours, or even 1 to 2 days, there will probably be reactive swelling of the nasal mucous membranes, and consequently the nasal passages may be more obstructed than before surgery.

POSTOPERATIVE MEDICATION

In most cases we prescribe a broad-spectrum oral antibiotic, usually penicillin or one of the cephalosporins, for at least 1 week. Although in most cases there may appear to be no pressing need for antibiotic coverage, our rationale for using antibiotics is as follows. Postoperatively there is a large wound surface with open mucosal areas measuring several square centimeters; consequently, there is always the danger of infection from the outside. The administration of antibiotics is therefore regarded as a prophylactic measure. There is no question about the administration of antibiotics when pus-filled cells were opened intraoperatively or when the disease process was either infectious or inflammatory or the complication of such a disease process or when an osteitis is present.

We do not prescribe postoperative antibiotics in mycotic infections of the paranasal sinuses unless there is concurrent massive bacterial superinfection, as is frequently encountered in the maxillary sinus, in the presence of fungus balls.

Systemic corticosteroids and antihistamines are not routinely prescribed. Corticosteroids are used only for the management of coincidental disease (e.g., asthma) when we are dealing with an inflammatory problem with polyp formation or in some cases of diffuse polypoid rhinosinusitis. In these situations we also administer antihistamines. In diffuse polypoid rhinosinusitis, corticosteroids are used in a rather desperate attempt to reduce the high recurrence rate somewhat and to promote wound healing.

An aqueous solution of beclomethasone nose drops or nasal spray (e.g., Beconase aqueous solution) has proved useful as a local agent, which we administer four to five times starting on the first postoperative day. In patients with marked polypoid disease, we prescribe corticosteroid nose drops for a period of at least 10 days, and frequently longer.

In some patients thick crusts tend to form in the operated area. The instillation of an oily nose drop will soften these crusts and make their removal easier. A satisfactory alternative is to have the patient sniff a homemade solution consisting of 1 tsp each of sugar, salt, and sodium bicarbonate dissolved in 240 mL warm water. If maxillary sinus endoscopy through the canine fossa produces mucosal swelling, the administration of an anti-inflammatory drug for a few days will usually be of benefit.

LOCAL POSTOPERATIVE CARE

Careful local postoperative care is an important component of our therapeutic concept, although it must be emphasized that the majority of operative cavities require little care. In some cases, however, the ultimate success of the surgical procedure depends largely on the postoperative care given.

On the first postoperative day, clots, secretions, and crusts should be removed carefully from the surgical site by suction. This must be done by the operating surgeon, because only he or she knows the precise extent of the procedure and those areas where special caution is necessary. When suctioning is performed on the first day, it is important that the suction tip be introduced under the middle turbinate and that secretions not be removed only from the nasal vestibule and the floor of the nose. Removal of secretions from the middle meatus prevents the formation of scabs and fibrin bridges that may contribute to later formation of synechia. These cleansing procedures must be performed carefully to avoid new trauma. In most cases this first suctioning can be performed without anesthesia and with the naked eye. In some cases, especially when the passages are narrow, the endoscope must be used and the suctioning must be performed under direct vision. Depending on patient sensitivity, a local anesthetic spray or pledgets may be required.

About 1 hour before the Merocel sponges are removed, a liquid solution such as beclomethasone should be dripped onto them to make the sponges more pliable. This reduces the risk of mucosal injury due to the irregular surfaces of the sponges.

When necessary, it may be possible to remove clots or tenacious secretions from the maxillary or frontal sinuses with a curved aspirator. To avoid fresh injury to the ostium, we prefer not to do this before the third postoperative day.

Nasal irrigation with saline or Ringer's solution is not routinely done during the first few postoperative days.

Suctioning and cleansing are performed again on the second and third postoperative days, and the patient is instructed to return after 1 week for follow up. At this time inspection with the endoscope is essential because it is usually possible to identify developing problems (e.g., synechia, ostial stenosis, disturbances of wound healing) or, most commonly, to observe an uncomplicated recovery (Fig 9–1). Also at this time, further visits can be scheduled. If there are no problems, we usually see the patient in 4 to 6 weeks, and decide then on the need for further visits. In problem cases, individual schedules must be developed.

The patient must be advised that the healing phase, particularly reepithelialization, will take at least 2 to 3 weeks, and may take as long as 6 weeks, or even longer in exceptional cases. During this time it is quite normal for some

A

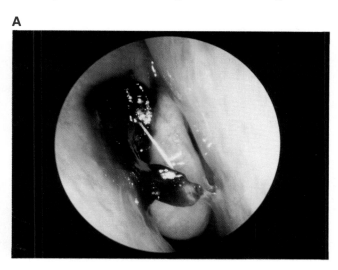

B

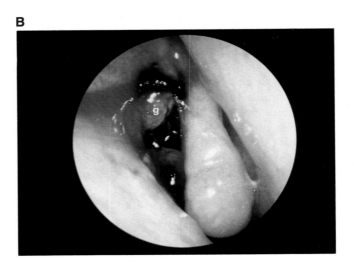

C

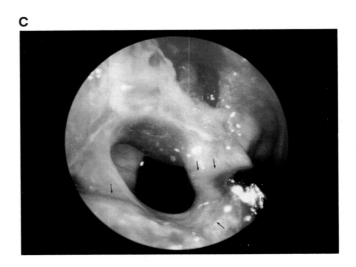

D

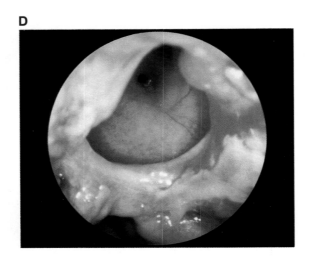

E

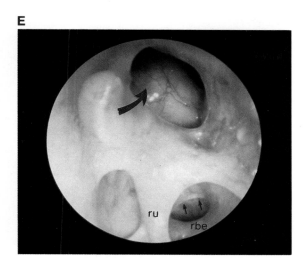

FIG 9–1.
A, view into the right side of a nose 3 days after endoscopic ethmoid surgery for mycotic sinusitis. The entrance into the middle meatus is covered with crusts. **B,** after removal of the crusts, some granulation tissue is found immediately below the insertion of the middle turbinate. The ethmoid cavity behind it is already healing nicely. *g* = granulation tissue. **C,** after the wound secretions are suctioned, a good view of the ostium of the maxillary sinus can be obtained. On the floor of the maxillary sinus, there are still some inspissated secretions, mixed with old coagulum. Note that in spite of the wound surfaces, the mucociliary transport already functions over a considerable area (*arrows* indicate the paths of the secretions from the ostium of the maxillary sinus and from the frontal recess). **D,** view into the maxillary sinus after aspiration of the wound secretions. The mucosa is still edematous and swollen but healing well. Note that the posterior rim of the ostium of the maxillary sinus was not traumatized but that the ostium was enlarged anteriorly at the expense of the fontanelles. The more firmly adherent fibrin deposits have not been removed yet. **E,** view at an endoscopic checkup 6 weeks after surgery. Note the patent passage into the frontal sinus through the enlarged frontal recess (*large arrow*). The posterior wall of the recess and its normal mucosa can be readily seen. The *thin arrows* point to a small anterior ethmoidal artery in the area of the lateral sinus. The mucosa has returned to normal in all areas. *ru* = remnants of the uncinate process; *rbe* = remnants of the ethmoidal bulla.

secretions to appear and for crusts to be expelled during sneezing or after blowing the nose. In severe polyposis, it may take several weeks before the maxillary and frontal sinuses revert to normal completely. For this reason, it makes little sense to do a repeat x-ray study in less than 6 to 8 weeks. Because the operative field can usually be well seen with the nasal endoscopes, we do not obtain postoperative x-ray films routinely, but reserve these for problem cases and complications.

POSTOPERATIVE PROBLEMS AND COMPLICATIONS

The nasal mucous membranes in some patients may respond to the minimal surgical trauma during the first few postoperative hours or days with such marked reactive mucosal engorgement that nasal breathing is initially more

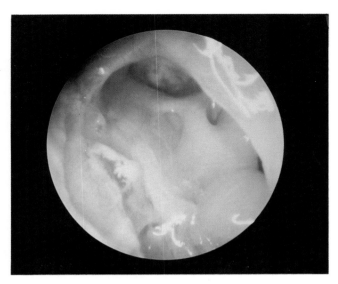

FIG 9–2.
In this patient, the mucosa shows no healing tendency 2 months after an endoscopic procedure for severe polypoid ethmoidal disease. The patient complained continuously about mucopurulent secretions, which reached the pharynx, and about a feeling of fullness. The poor healing tendency was probably the result of an underlying osteitis. After 10 days of IV therapy with ciprofloxacin and a combination of cortisone and antihistamine twice daily, orally, the symptoms rapidly regressed and the mucosa returned to normal.

obstructed than it was preoperatively. The patient must be told in advance that this is not a complication and that it should be considered entirely normal.

Even a minor crust occasionally can give rise to significant symptoms. As a precursor to epithelialization, these scabs or crusts consist of inspissated secretions and fibrin deposits. They can solidify, and may fill the entire surgical area like a cast. They must be removed with the greatest care so as not to cause additional injury or renewed bleeding. Even a tiny (1 to 2 mm) crust, if located at the entrance to the middle meatus, and particularly if situated in a transverse direction, may give the patient the impression of complete respiratory obstruction, even though there is practically no interference with the air stream. It is always astonishing how the removal of such a tiny crust leads to subjective improvement in nasal respiration.

In patients with diffuse polypoid rhinosinusitis, granular or polypoid changes frequently recur in the mucous membranes within a few postoperative days. Occasionally edematous polyps reappear in the ethmoidal sinus on the first or second postoperative day. These should be promptly removed. It is often frustrating to see how in spite of intensive and expensive local management, removal of crusts and secretions, and application of corticosteroids, the diffuse mucosal changes characteristic of this disease regress only extremely slowly, and in some cases may even worsen during therapy.

We must be able to identify those persistent granulating changes, hypersecretion, and disturbances of wound healing that occur in those cases with osteitis of an underlying bony structure. Clinically this is characterized by a finely granular, weepy mucosal surface with frequently smeary, purulent secretions and occasionally small edematous inflammatory polyps in this area (Fig 9–2). These cases usually require prolonged and careful local management and the administration of a specific high-dose, long-term, sometimes intravenous antibiotic regimen. In these cases, combination therapy of antibiotics and corticosteroids is frequently successful.

With the Messerklinger technique, the enlarged ostium of the maxillary sinus in the middle meatus shows surprisingly little inclination toward stenosis (see Chapter 11). To traumatize the ostium as little as possible postoperatively, we do not routinely irrigate the maxillary sinus, and suction retained secretions only when they spontaneously liquefy after the third or fourth postoperative day. If the maxillary sinus has been diseased for months or even years, it may take many days or weeks before ciliary activity fully returns to normal and before mucus of normal consistency is produced.

SERIOUS COMPLICATIONS DURING AFTERCARE

We used to instill antibiotic and corticosteroid ointments into the middle meatus; however, in recent years we have ceased this practice. Instillation of such ointments has no advantages for wound healing or prevention of synechia and crusts. Within minutes or hours after instillation, the ointment is transported into the nasopharynx, where it produces an unpleasant taste. In some patients with recurrent problems, we found remnants of the ointment in obstructed sections of the ethmoidal sinus, although there was no evidence that the ointment was responsible for the recurrence of disease. The occasional observation of fungal growth on top of such encapsulated ointment has further induced us to abandon this practice.

We are aware of several cases in which the ointment was introduced into the orbit, where it produced serious complications (e.g., persistent diplopia). In addition to inadvertent direct instillation of ointment into the orbit through an unrecognized perforation of the lamina papyracea, it is also possible for ointment to penetrate into the orbit through the site of a minor prolapse of orbital fat that was missed intraoperatively. Such cases have also contributed to our discontinuing the practice of instilling ointments into the surgical field.

We have also seen several cases in which instillation of antimycotic ointment into the middle meatus or the maxillary sinus was followed by extremely painful and persistent granulomatous infiltrates into the soft tissues of the cheeks. Apparently the antibiotic ointments reached the soft tissues through the openings in the canine fossa, which were created by the insertion of the maxillary sinus trocar. In those cases where maxillary sinus endoscopy is performed as part of the surgical procedure, we instill antimycotic preparations, if at all, only after the fifth or sixth postoperative day, by which time it can be assumed with reasonable certainty that the trocar openings have completely closed.

Foreign substances such as cotton pledgets or Merocel sponges left in the operative field may lead to serious complications. All pledgets or sponges introduced into the nose must be marked with a long suture to assure their recognition and removal. When a sponge is left intentionally for some time, the thread attached to it should be taped to the patient's cheek to prevent the sponge from advancing into the pharynx and to alert the aftercare team of its presence. When a sponge is to be left in place for a prolonged period, the amount of tissue reaction to the sponge may be decreased by suturing a thin sheet of Silastic sheeting over the sponge.

DISCHARGE INSTRUCTIONS

For at least 1 week postoperatively, the patient should not engage in vigorous sports or any general activities that may lead to sudden hypertension (e.g., bending, lifting heavy objects, sauna, excessive alcohol intake, sunbathing). The patient must be made aware of the phases of wound healing, and should understand that reepithelialization may take several weeks and that the presence of secretions and crust formation are normal during this period.

The patient should have reasonable expectations, and must be made to understand that the operation does not immunize against future upper respiratory tract infections. Colds may very well develop, with nasal and paranasal sinus symptoms and even episodes of sinusitis, which must be treated appropriately. The incidence and severity of such infections should, however, be appreciably less than before surgery. They should be of shorter duration, and most important, should not become chronic.

Patients with diffuse polypoid rhinosinusitis with massive tissue eosinophilia (nonallergic rhinosinusitis with esosinophilia, or NARES syndrome), aspirin-sensitive asthma intolerance, asthma, and cystic fibrosis, should be informed that surgery may sometimes considerably and dramatically improve their symptoms. However, with our understanding of these diseases today, no type of surgery can offer a definitive cure. Intermittent or permanent continued medical therapy, both local and systemic, may be necessary until research can find a better solution to these problems.

10 Results

Because of the large number of indications for the Messerklinger technique of functional endoscopic sinus surgery (Table 10–1), no single, unified statistic is capable of accurately representing the results of this technique; rather, the results must be examined on the basis of the disease entities treated.

Any assessment of the results of surgery is further complicated by the lack of criteria that can be applied to provide a truly objective measurement of postoperative "success." In many indications, such as headache, facial pressure, postnasal discharge, or frequent or protracted colds with obstructed nasal breathing, the assessor is almost totally dependent on the patient's subjective evaluation. Rhinomanometry has not proved useful in our hands as either a determinant for surgery or a measure of successful outcome. Frequently even after extensive sinus surgery with preservation of the middle turbinate, patients show the same rhinomanometric curves postoperatively as preoperatively, even though the subjective symptoms reported by the patient are significantly improved or even eliminated and endoscopy reveals normal mucous membranes.

Because we can examine the most remote corners of the paranasal sinus system and the lateral wall of the nose postoperatively with the endoscope, it becomes apparent that objective evaluation of the outcome is also difficult (Fig 10–1). We have seen a number of patients who were free of symptoms for years after a surgical procedure, yet whose mucous membranes were far from "normal" (Fig 10–2). One may find mild inflammatory changes, polypoid thickening, crusts, and increased secretions in patients with sinubronchial syndrome or asthma with aspirin intolerance who postoperatively report significant improvement in nasal symptoms and even complete disappearance of asthma. Many of these patients had been corticosteroid-dependent preop-

TABLE 10–1

Spectrum of Frequent Indications for Functional Endoscopic Sinus Surgery

Polypoid sinusitis (60%)	Symptomatic retention cysts
Chronic and acute recurring infections of all sinuses	Orbital complications
	Sinus mycoses
Nasal obstruction	Persisting complaints after Caldwell-Luc
Headaches	and fenestration operations
Pressure feelings	Tubal dysfunctions
Postnasal discharge	Adjuvant surgery to allergy treatment
Epiphora	Antrochoanal polyps
Anosmia	Mucoviscidosis
Mucoceles of all sinuses	Sinubronchial syndrome/asthma

eratively, but were able to reduce or discontinue the steroid regimen and consequently noted significant improvement in the quality of their life.

On the other hand, some patients whose mucous membranes appear to be perfectly normal postoperatively and whose ostia are all free and patent still complain of a variety of persistent problems for which no anatomic basis can be found. In these patients, unrealistic expectations may conflict with reality. For this reason, we explain to patients in detail that the surgical procedure will not protect them from future colds and that sinusitis may even develop again.

All this shows that it is difficult to give percentages of objective postoperative improvement and to develop meaningful statistics. For example, how should the results of surgery be classified in a patient whose asthma has disappeared postoperatively, whose nasal respiration is improved, but whose mucous membrane is abnormal? (Fig 10–2). Should success be rated as 100% based on improvement in clinical symptoms? Or only 60%, on the basis of endoscopic findings? In contrast, how should results be rated in the patient whose mucous membranes have become completely normal but who still complains of a variety of inexplicable and unclassifiable residual problems or if preoperatively and postoperatively "nasal polyps" are considered as one disease entity? How can the results of different surgeons, perhaps using different techniques, be compared, when one of the raters does not use an endoscope postoperatively and thus cannot see the residual changes and relies entirely on the patient's clinical symptoms? These are just some of a variety of unresolved questions that indicate the difficulty in gathering statistics and in comparing the results of different authors.

In our postoperative assessment, we ask patients to indicate a percent improvement (see later discussion); we then attempt to relate this subjective change to endoscopic and radiologic findings , and express these findings as a percentage. The statistics presented clearly still contain a significant subjective component.

During 1986 and 1987 we evaluated the results in more than 500 patients who had undergone functional endoscopic sinus surgery performed with the Messerklinger technique from 8 months to 10 years previously and in whom the surgical indications encompassed a wide spectrum. In all patients a diagnostic nasal endoscopy was performed, a careful history taken, and a detailed questionnaire completed by the patients and then evaluated by a third person.

The various surgical procedures that had been performed without much success in these patients before functional endoscopic sinus surgery included frequent repeated maxillary irrigations or insertion of indwelling tubes for drainage; fenestration or radical surgery, some multiple and bilateral (n = 82); septoplasty (54); and multiple previous "standard" polypectomies (69). The large number of patients whose symptoms were not improved by fenestration or Caldwell-Luc procedures is noteworthy. More than 10% of patients had undergone one or more septoplasties. It was not possible to accurately determine the number of patients who had undergone partial resection of the middle or inferior turbinates. Most patients could not remember whether turbinate resection was performed as part of another procedure. Even endoscopic examination could not fully confirm these reports.

Independent of the extent and severity of the original disease process, the best postoperative results were achieved in those patients in whom anatomic variations could be identified as responsible for the underlying problems. Particularly good results were obtained in those patients who were operated on because of sinugenic headaches; 88% reported that their symptoms had either

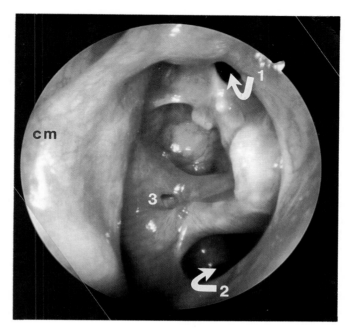

FIG 10–1.
View into a left ethmoidal sinus 1 year after surgery. The path to the maxillary and frontal sinuses is free (*curved arrows 1 and 2*). The mucosa is unremarkable everywhere. At *3,* it is still possible to see the somewhat scarred opening into the ground lamella that was made to inspect the posterior ethmoidal sinus. Note that no attempt had been made to create a large and smooth operative cavity. Only the important pathologic changes were corrected. *1* = to maxillary sinus; *2* = to frontal sinus; *3* = scarred opening into the ground lamella; *cm* = concha media.

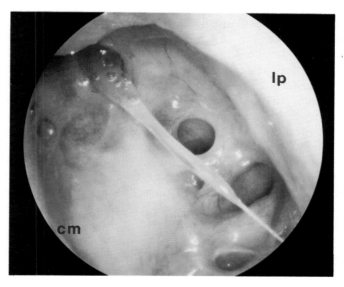

FIG 10–2.
Abnormal mucosa, postoperatively, in a left middle meatus. For details, see text. *s* = septum; *cm* = concha media.

disappeared or were significantly improved. Good results were also obtained in mycotic infections of the paranasal sinuses, although only when the mycoses were noninvasive.

Allergies had no statistically significant effect on the postoperative results. Allergic rhinosinusitis is not a primary indication for an endoscopic surgical procedure. However, when an endoscopic procedure was performed as an adjuvant measure to manage obstruction in the middle meatus and ethmoid complex, the results were clearly better in those patients who had already shown some improvement with antiallergic medical management.

Another important factor in the success rate was whether the endoscopic procedure was the first surgical intervention. When a number of other procedures had been performed previously, the endoscopic surgery was much more difficult, as was postoperative assessment by both the patient and the surgeon. It was sometimes impossible to distinguish between residual complaints after the Messerklinger technique and those complaints that persisted from a previous procedure (e.g., previous Caldwell-Luc procedure).

Patient reports showed a pattern in which certain symptoms disappeared. Patients consistently reported that headaches or feeling of fullness or pressure between the eyes disappeared immediately (within the first few hours) after the endoscopic procedure. Tearing also stopped within hours, or at most within 1 to 2 days. Postnasal drip, a symptom most patients found particularly bothersome, almost always stopped within the first operative day.

A number of patients reported improvement in nasal breathing while still on the operating table. During the first few postoperative days there was again "partial obstruction" of the nose due to reactive swelling of the mucosa. In most cases the feeling of obstructed nasal breathing disappeared completely in 1 to 2 weeks, or only occasionally by 6 weeks. In individual patients, increased secretions and crusting also lasted up to 6 weeks.

Our worst results were obtained in those patients with diffuse polypoid rhinosinopathy. Of the 500 patients studied, 246 had more or less massive polyposis. In 64 of these patients diffuse polypoid rhinosinopathy was manifested by massive inflammatory, primarily eosinophilic, infiltration, that is, nonallergic rhinosinusitis with eosinophilia (NARES syndrome). Of this group, slightly more than 18% had recurrent symptoms after only a short time. In most cases, a few weeks of improvement were followed by increasing nasal obstruction and polypoid mucous membrane changes. Local and systemic corticosteroid therapy produced variable and unpredictable results in these patients. In some cases, repeated endoscopic procedures were followed, surprisingly, by extended periods (even years) with no symptoms. This happened even though the second and third endoscopic procedures were no more radical than the initial operation.

When we realized that diffuse, polypoid rhinosinopathy (NARES syndrome) probably represented a unique disease entity, and because we were disappointed with the results of our conservative surgical procedure, we started using a radical approach, with resection of the middle turbinate, external approaches, total sphenoethmoidectomies, and so forth. We found, however, that these radical techniques did not yield statistically demonstrable better long-term results than the more conservative endoscopic techniques. On the contrary, patients had more postoperative problems after radical surgery.

It is our impression that diffuse polypoid rhinosinopathy is an idiopathic generalized disease of the entire mucous membrane of the upper (and possibly the lower) airway for which there is at present no rational therapy. Management of this disease clearly requires more than surgery (of whatever type). Ultimate therapy will probably be pharmacologic.

We must differentiate diffuse polypoid rhinosinopathy from persistent polypoid mucosal swelling with tenacious and purulent secretions that can be attributed to limited or more extensive osteitis or periostitis. In this case, long-term specific antibiotic therapy usually yields excellent improvement or even complete recovery.

Another largely unresolved problem is paranasal sinus mucosa that appears to be essentially normal postoperatively, yet has not significantly improved. Patients, primarily those with bronchial asthma or the aspirin-sensitive asthma (ASA) triad, still produce a highly viscous, rubbery secretion that cannot be completely removed by ciliary action from the paranasal sinuses and from the recesses of the ethmoidal sinuses (Fig 10–3). Mucosal biopsy specimens show a slight increase in goblet cells, which is insufficient to explain the increased production of mucus. The mucosal glands appear normal on light microscopy. The cause of this disorder is unknown.

Symptomatic therapy with inhaled mucolytic agents and a variety of nasal sprays occasionally produces significant improvement, but in most cases is totally ineffective. Occasionally the secretions are so viscous that they cannot be removed with suction, and a Blakesley forceps must be used.

Radical surgical procedures are not helpful in these patients either. To perform radical surgery in the face of essentially normal macroscopic conditions is of questionable benefit. In some severe cases we have performed a fenestration of the inferior meatus to facilitate the removal of the secretions by gravity or at least to establish an opening into the maxillary sinus for the aspirator.

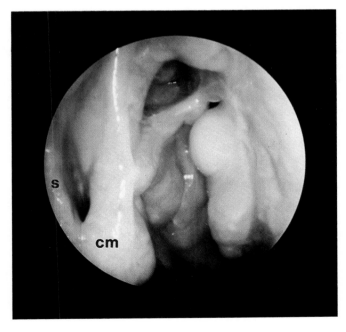

FIG 10–3.
Tenacious secretions are shown coming from the frontal sinus in a patient with otherwise normal mucosa. For details, see text. *lp* = lamina papyracea; *cm* = concha media.

The most unfavorable outlook for a surgical procedure is the combination of a diffuse polypoid rhinosinopathy and ASA sensitivity, with a long history of bronchial asthma (ASA triad) and viscous paranasal sinus secretions combined with a number of previous procedures that have destroyed the anatomic landmarks and led to extensive scar formation.

The results of examination and survey of 500 patients, who were reexamined in 1986 and 1987 (follow-up time 8 months to 10 years), are as follows. Eighty five percent (425 patients) reported good or very good results. Six percent (30) were satisfied with the results. Four percent (21) reported only moderate success; and another 4% (23) reported no improvement of symptoms postoperatively, although none of these reported any aggravation of symptoms. In one patient, 1 year after the endoscopic surgery asthma appeared for the first time, but no causal relationship between this event and the surgery could be established.

The results in patients with asthma are also encouraging. Slightly more than 60% of patients with intrinsic bronchial asthma reported impressive and persistent improvement in symptoms postoperatively, and these improvements were documented by improved FEV_1 (forced expiratory volume in 1 minute) and reduced drug use. Twenty percent showed only transient, subjective improvement not supported by FEV_1 changes, and 10% reported no improvement in asthma symptoms. It was surprising that the duration of asthma symptoms preoperatively bore no relationship to postoperative results.

Although it is clinically obvious that endoscopic surgical management of disease of the lateral nasal wall in patients with bronchial asthma can produce beneficial results, there are no criteria to predict in which patients, to what extent, and for how long such improvements will occur. Despite this, our results and clinical experience encourage us to operate not only in cases of massive nasal and paranasal sinus diseases but also when the changes are relatively limited.

Because a number of the 500 patients in our study had undergone surgery up to 10 years previously, and because at that time patients were not routinely queried about loss of sense of smell, nor were tests of smell performed, we have no statistically meaningful data on this topic. On a purely historical basis, about 23% of the 500 patients indicated that they had some decrease in their sense of smell preoperatively. Many of these patients also indicated that there was a definite improvement in this parameter postoperatively. In most cases, no precise, retrospective measurement of either loss or improvement in sense of smell was possible.

11 Postoperative Problems and Complications

SYNECHIA

Synechia are most likely to develop when opposing wound surfaces are created during surgery (e.g., when the head of the middle turbinate is injured during work on the anterior ethmoidal sinus). This can occur easily when the passage into the middle meatus is very narrow (e.g., when the middle meatus has a paradoxical bend) or if the head of the middle turbinate is very large and is tightly pressed against the lateral nasal wall. The best prophylaxis against the development of synechia is scrupulous attention to atraumatic surgery and prevention of injury to the mucosa of the middle turbinate.

Opposing wound surfaces can be created during partial resection of a concha bullosa, even though the distance to the lateral nasal wall after the lateral lamella of the concha has been removed is usually great enough to prevent the formation of adhesions. If however, the remaining medial lamella of the concha bullosa is unstable because it was fractured during the procedure, synechia can form at the insertion of the turbinate, which may scar the free part of the turbinate to the lateral nasal wall over a period of several weeks or months.

In 8% (43 of 500) of our patients at follow-up examination we observed synechia of various sizes between the head of the middle turbinate and the lateral nasal wall (Fig 11–1).

The presence of synechia does not necessarily mean that the patient will have recurrence of symptoms. Only 20% (8 of 43) of patients in whom we found synechia had persistent or recurrent symptoms that could be attributed exclusively to the synechia. These problems usually appeared when the synechia constricted the entrance to the middle meatus or closed off parts of the ethmoidal sinus, causing retention of secretions and narrowing of the ostia. If there is scar formation that directly obstructs the ostium of the maxillary sinus, symptoms return quite quickly.

In some patients, there may be only a thin anterior synechia that impedes the entrance to the middle meatus (see Fig 11–1). This may be enough to create the sensation of severely obstructed nasal breathing, even though the nasal cavity is completely patent and the ethmoid process behind the synechia is entirely normal. This observation emphasizes the importance of unobstructed aeration of the middle meatus for the subjective feeling of free nasal airflow.

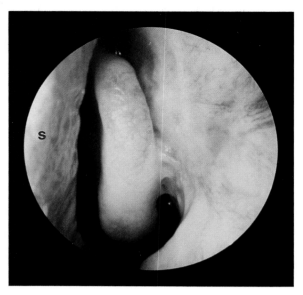

FIG 11–1.
A sheet of adhesions are visible between the left middle turbinate and the lamina papyracea. *s* = septum.

Synechia are easily identified and managed endoscopically. They are divided and the excessive scar tissue resected, and a small piece of Silastic or other type of stent is inserted for a few days. This minor procedure usually eliminates the synechia.

The recurrence of synechia cannot always be prevented. In some cases we have seen adhesions appear after many years of complete freedom from problems. Apparently these late adhesions developed after a viral infection with concomitant epithelial lesions. Resection of the middle turbinate is not usually indicated, because synechia may still develop medially, toward the septum, and can then obstruct the rima olfactoria. Furthermore, the additional trauma (pain, bleeding) and the removal of key anatomic landmarks are usually unjustified.

OVERLOOKED DISEASE

Massively diseased ethmoidal cells or fissures, if overlooked at the time of endoscopic (or other) surgery, can be the reason for persistent or recurring problems. Such cells were either incorrectly diagnosed or overlooked during surgery because of increased bleeding or, for example, uncertainty of the surgeon about the ethmoidal topography. This and other postoperative problems can be readily identified and appropriately managed endoscopically (Figs 11–2 and 11–3).

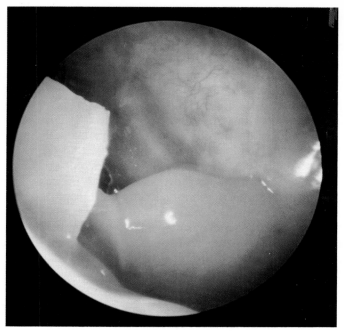

FIG 11–2.
On closer examination, it became evident that the "retention cysts" were actually two bone fragments extending from the floor of the sphenoid sinus into its lumen that were covered by a purulent exudate. These sequestered bone spicules were probably displaced into the lumen of the sinus at the time the anterior wall of the sinus was perforated (fractured inward) and that then became necrotic. After removal of these sequestra, the patient's recovery was uneventful.

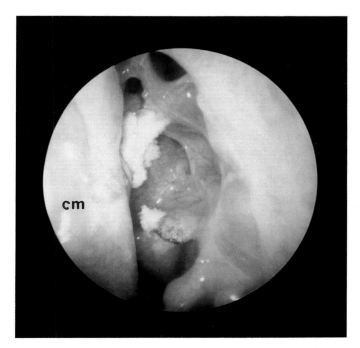

FIG 11–3.
Left ethmoid cavity 6 months after surgery for polypoid disease. The mucosa is more or less unremarkable. There is fungal growth on crusts following excessive use of cortisone-containing nasal spray. *cm* = concha media.

Stenosis of Maxillary Sinus Ostium

The percentage of problems attributable to stenosis of an enlarged maxillary sinus ostium was surprisingly small in our series. Only eight of 500 patients (<2%) had a functional stenosis. In one patient stenosis developed on three consecutive occasions despite an apparently correct surgical technique.

Reepithelialization of the edges of a surgically enlarged ostium apparently is rapid. One explanation for this may be that the transportation of secretions from the maxillary sinus once again takes place through the natural ostium and that this contributes to the rapid healing process. Furthermore, the Messerklinger technique prevents a complete circumferential lesion of the ostium, because the ostium is enlarged only at the expense of the anterior fontanelle. If the posterior fontanelle is also enlarged (e.g., if there is an accessory ostium in that area), the result is an ostium 10 by 6 to 8 mm in diameter, which provides adequate ventilation and drainage even if it should shrink to half this size. In our experience, a diameter of 3 mm is sufficient to provide a physiologic functioning ostium for the maxillary sinus.

POSTOPERATIVE BLEEDING

In 11 patients there was such severe intraoperative or immediate postoperative hemorrhage that nasal packing became necessary. In one of these 11 patients a posterior pack (Bellocq) was required. This was also the only patient in our entire series of more than 9,000 to date in whom a transfusion became necessary, which was partially the result of a missed coagulopathy.

In the ten other cases a repeat endoscopic procedure had to be performed because bleeding obstructed the view during the initial surgery. During the last few years, the number of cases in which bleeding forced cessation of the procedure has dropped to less than 1%.

ADDITIONAL COMPLICATIONS

In the 500 patients in our study, additional complications were seen. In nine patients there was a definite injury to the lamina papyracea and to the periorbital area, with prolapse of orbital fat. Three of these patients had edema of the eyelid on the first postoperative day, and two patients had a hematoma at the inner canthus. In none of these patients was there any additional complication, such as diplopia or infection of the orbital contents.

Other complications included soft tissue infiltration after sinoscopy (five patients) and "forgotten" Merocel sponge (one patient).

AVOIDING COMPLICATIONS

Intraoperative Bleeding

Normally bleeding is not a problem when local and topical anesthesia are used. The best way to prevent intraoperative hemorrhage is to prepare the patient carefully (control of hypertension, good sedation, topical and local anesthesia) and use a careful, atraumatic surgical technique. Hasty procedures should be avoided in acute inflammation, and medical treatment given until optimal preoperative conditions are present.

Bleeding is almost never from an isolated, single vessel, but is usually a generalized oozing from the edges of the mucous membranes at the site of resection. This type of bleeding is more likely to be bothersome when one is operating on a patient with an acute inflammatory problem with corresponding hyperemia. In most cases this type of bleeding can be stopped with repeated application of tetracaine (Pontocaine) and epinephrine–soaked cotton sponges. The sponges are introduced into the middle meatus under gentle pressure and left in place for 2 to 3 minutes. It is then usually possible to continue the procedure without undue difficulty. If it is necessary to keep the sponges in place longer, the surgeon can operate on the other side in the interim and not waste time waiting. Measurements have shown that the average blood loss after bilateral surgery is less than 30 mL (our one patient who required a transfusion is not included in the calculation of this average loss).

The surgeon must always follow the principle that when exposure is seriously limited by hemorrhage the procedure must be discontinued. It is safer to operate again another day than to create an iatrogenic complication. The best feature of endoscopic surgery with the Messerklinger technique is good visibility and the ability to know at all times one's precise location in respect to the various components of the ethmoid system.

Bipolar cautery forceps can be helpful when bleeding is from an individual vessel. This is most likely around the ostium of the maxillary sinus or at the insertion of the middle turbinate. For capillary oozing, the placement of fingernail sized pieces of Oxycel over the bleeding area has proved useful. Oxycel adheres well to the underlying surface and controls the oozing effectively. Even bleeding from small squirting vessels can usually be controlled with an Oxycel pack. For this purpose, we place an appropriately shaped piece of Oxycel on a cotton applicator and hold it in place with gentle pressure with a pair of forceps. After 1 minute the cotton applicator is removed. The Oxycel usually adheres to the mucosa and stops the bleeding.

The posterior end of the middle turbinate is another place from which bleeding may originate. Because of its proximity to the sphenopalatine foramen and the mucosal vessels entering and leaving through this space, injury and hemorrhage can occur quite readily in this area. With the exception of an extensively pneumatized middle turbinate, the Messerklinger technique does not usually traumatize the area of the posterior end of the middle turbinate. On the other hand, when necessary the sphenopalatine foramen can be easily identified with the endoscope and any hemorrhage controlled with Oxycel and pressure.

Because all of the cellular septa are not removed routinely in the Messerklinger technique to create a standardized ethmoid cavity, the danger of injury to the anterior and posterior ethmoidal arteries is minimal. With the Messerklinger technique, it is not necessary to smooth the roof of the ethmoidal sinus with a diamond drill to "ideal" smoothness. If this were done, the thin bony covering of the vessels may be perforated and injury to the vessels may occur.

Bleeding from the anterior ethmoidal artery is generally not dramatic, and the pulsating vessel can usually be easily identified and managed. Tetracaine-epinephrine–soaked sponges are also useful when applied with gentle pressure and buttressed with Oxycel. Coagulation by cautery and placement of a silver clip are also effective. When required by the procedure, the anterior ethmoidal artery can usually be easily identified and avoided during the remainder of the procedure.

Retroorbital Hematoma

A severed anterior ethmoidal artery can produce one of the most dangerous complications in the entire field of ethmoidal surgery. This happens if the vessel retracts into the orbit and continues to bleed. The resulting periorbital or intraorbital hematoma can produce all of the dreaded orbital complications, including blindness. We have seen two cases of orbital hematoma due to injury to the anterior ethmoidal artery. Within a few seconds the eyeball protruded and became fixed. In such cases *the surgeon must be prepared to perform emergency decompression of the orbit to prevent blindness.*

This type of complication reemphasizes the advantages of operating with the patient under local anesthesia. The fundus and vision can be immediately checked, and the patient can give precise information about visual field changes. With the patient under general anesthesia, precious time may be lost in deciding whether orbital decompression is necessary while waiting for the patient to wake up so that the visual fields and acuity of vision can be assessed and fundoscopic examination performed.

To determine whether decompression is indicated, it is helpful to have diagnostic ultrasound equipment available to locate the hematoma. The surgeon can then determine where the hematoma is, in which direction it is expanding (periorbitally, intraorbitally, retrobulbarly), and the degree of displacement, stretching, and flexing of the optic nerve. A periorbital hemorrhage between the lamina papyracea and the periorbital area only rarely produces visual field defects or visual problems. Both of our cases were of this type, and required no further surgical intervention.

When the slightest evidence of visual field loss or obvious loss of vision occurs, immediate action is necessary. It is the recommendation of our ophthalmologists that the first step should be an immediate lateral canthotomy and adjacent opening of the orbital septum (in the area of the lower lid). This allows the periorbital fat to move anteriorly, thereby decreasing the intraorbital pressure and the pressure on the optic nerve and optic vessels. After these initial emergency measures, decompression of the orbit can be carried out, with identification and control of the site of bleeding. An external approach above the eyebrow may be the technique of choice.

If an intraorbital or periorbital hematoma has been demonstrated and visual loss or impairment of the visual field has occurred, medical management with only diuretics, mannitol infusion, and corticosteroid administration is not recommended.

The less experienced surgeon should never try to operate around the ethmoid roof, the lamina papyracea, or the posterior ethmoidal and sphenoidal areas blindly or by palpation. Reports of cases in which serious complications have occurred (e.g., serious orbital lesions, perforation of the roof of the ethmoidal sinus, lesions to the optic nerve) have one element in common: the procedure was done with the patient under general anesthesia, there was bleeding, and visibility was not good. Hence, *if you cannot see, Stop!*

TABLE 11–1

Severe Complications Since 1976
(More Than 8,000 Patients)

CSF leaks	4
Pneumatocephalus	1
Intraorbital bleeding	2
Meningitis	0
Partial loss of vision	
Diplopia	0
Blindness	0
Fatalities	0
Stenosis of the nasolacrimal duct	0

SEVERE COMPLICATIONS

All of the serious complications that occurred in more than 8,000 patients operated on since 1976 are listed in Table 11–1. Intraorbital hemorrhage has been discussed.

We know of four cases of iatrogenic cerebrospinal fluid (CSF) fistulas. Two of these patients had recurrent nasal polyps and had undergone several previous operations. During the endoscopic procedure, the ethmoidal anatomy was difficult to identify because of the previous surgery. The insertion of the middle turbinate was missing, and there was extensive scarring and many adhesions. As determined retrospectively, the dura was injured in both of these patients at its typical weak spot, the roof of the ethmoid at the place where the anterior ethmoidal artery exits through the lateral lamina of the cribriform plate. Some of the polyps were adherent to the dura at this point, and the attempt to remove them apparently caused the dura to tear.

The third patient's history revealed a basal skull fracture sustained several years previously, although on tomography no evidence of any bony abnormality or defect of the roof of the ethmoid was found. In this patient the perforation was at the level of the insertion of the ground lamella at the roof of the ethmoid in the posterior aspect of the lateral sinus. It seems likely that a preexisting bony defect from the previous skull fracture was hidden by scar tissue. In this case, the dural defect was repaired at the same endoscopic procedure. A small piece of appropriately shaped lyophilized dura was placed between the injured dura and the base of the skull. A medially based mucosal flap, from the lateral surface of the middle turbinate, was then pasted over the area with fibrin adhesive. Oxycel was packed in the area under light pressure, and the patient was confined to bed for 5 days with strict instructions not to blow his nose.

In one of the two other cases the CSF fistula was clearly visible during the procedure. Because it was small, it was covered with a mucous membrane flap and tamponaded with an Oxycel sponge. The hoped for spontaneous closure did not take place, and a few days later an external, transethmoidal closure was performed. No further problems ensued.

In the other patient there was no evidence for a dural defect either intraoperatively or during the first 2 postoperative days. On the third postoperative day, after blowing his nose, the patient developed increasingly severe headaches. A skull x-ray film showed a marked internal and external pneumocephalus. The CSF fistula was identified by means of a fluorescein study, then closed from outside through the ethmoidal sinus. There were no persistent complications.

In the fourth case, immediate-onset meningitis developed postoperatively, which was controlled medically. The iatrogenic dural defect was closed endoscopically.

None of our patients developed diplopia, transient loss of vision, or blindness. There have been no deaths related to the endoscopic procedures.

Optic Nerve Injury

Although we have never seen an injury to the optic nerve or to the internal carotid artery, we are aware from the literature and from personal communications from our colleagues that this has happened during an endoscopic procedure. When these cases are studied, it becomes apparent that the injuries to the optic nerve were not in the sphenoidal sinus, where all surgeons are acutely aware of this possibility, but occurred in the area of the posterior ethmoidal sinus (See Chapters 2 and 8). It is critical, therefore, to keep the anatomy and the anatomic variations of this area in mind. One must be particularly aware of the possible existence of the Onodi cells (see Chapter 2), which may extend the boundaries of the posterior ethmoid laterally and superiorly of the sphenoidal sinus. If the Onodi cells are extensively pneumatized, not only the optic nerve but also the internal carotid artery may bulge into the lateral or superior wall of these enlarged posterior ethmoidal cells. If the bone is extremely thin or dehiscent over these bulges, the danger of iatrogenic injury is acute.

In the presence of large Onodi cells, one must keep in mind that the sphenoidal sinus is not a direct extension of the Onodi cells in a posterolateral direction. The sphenoidal sinus must be looked for medially and inferiorly. In the sphenoidal sinus proper, any sharp or forceful removal of the mucous membranes from the lateral wall, roof, and posterior wall of the cavity must stop unless the surgeon is absolutely certain that there are no bony dehiscences or dangerous anatomic variants present.

Bony septa in the sphenoidal sinus should be removed only with extreme care (if at all) and only after careful study of the computed tomography (CT) scans, which must be present in the operating room. These septa frequently do not run medially, and they may insert into a thin bony shell over the optic nerve or carotid artery. This bony shell can be easily fractured during an attempt to remove the septa, and the optic nerve or the carotid artery may be injured.

The lamina papyracea may be very thin also over the medial aspect of the apex of the orbit. The surgeon should be able to distinguish between periorbital fat and diseased mucous membrane. An injury to or transsection of the optic nerve in the orbit directly behind the bulb is evidence for complete disregard of the Messerklinger technique and ignorance of the anatomy of this area.

The most dramatic case we know of is that of a patient in whom both optic nerves were cut and resected within the orbit immediately behind the bulb. This case was described in the operative note as a "functional endoscopic procedure." The procedure actually performed—radical surgery with resection of the middle and superior turbinate and part of the inferior turbinate—clearly was not "functional." Many of the complications attributed to the endoscopic procedure must, in reality, be attributed to the surgeon. Functional endoscopic sinus surgery and endonasal surgery using an endoscope are not necessarily identical.

Carotid Artery Injury

We have never been faced with a hemorrhage from the carotid artery. We suspect that if the injury is punctate, the immediate application of an Oxycel sponge under pressure may control the hemorrhage. If the injury is substantial with profuse hemorrhage, possible emergency measures to be considered include tight packing, manual compression of the common carotid artery in the neck against the cervical vertebrae on the affected side, and ligation of this vessel. Extensive neurosurgical exploration may or may not be able to prevent a life-threatening situation or severe permanent central nervous system damage. No predictions can be made for the individual case. The success should depend on the availability of adequate collateral circulation through the circle of Willis, immediate availability of suitable blood in sufficient quantity, and the immediate availability of a skilled neurosurgeon. We know of one case in which the carotid hemorrhage was controlled transiently, but the patient died of complications within a few days.

Other intracranial lesions we have heard about include penetration into the ventricular system with an instrument, and an iatrogenic lesion of the communicating artery between the anterior cerebral arteries with ensuing intracerebral hemorrhage.

TRAINING

The surgical aspects of the Messerklinger technique require solid training and an excellent knowledge of the anatomy of the lateral nasal wall and all its variations. The technique carries all the risks and dangers of any type of endonasal ethmoidal surgery, but when used for the appropriate indications and performed skillfully by an experienced surgeon, the Messerklinger technique carries only a minimal incidence of complications.

None of the various endoscopic schools has claimed that their technique is an easier or safer route to the ethmoidal sinus. The endoscope is not the end, but a means to functional therapy.

There are many excellent opportunities today to learn the endoscopic technique. Training lenses and small video cameras make it possible for the trainee to directly follow the diagnostic and therapeutic manipulations. The actual surgical procedure should be attempted only after having performed both diagnostic and therapeutic procedures many times (we recommend at least 20–30) on cadavers or anatomic preparations. Only in this way can true familiarity with the anatomy and the anatomic variations of the area be gained.

The endoscopist must become thoroughly familiar with the endoscope through a number of diagnostic procedures, and progress to surgical procedures only after facility in the management of the instrument and complete familiarity with the anatomic structures have been obtained. The beginner should never start with a difficult case, such as a patient who has had previous surgery or a patient with severe recurrent polyposis or scar formation that distorts the anatomy. Whoever wishes to perform endoscopic surgery must be willing to practice the same careful, atraumatic technique as for stapes surgery, and must also be prepared to assume the sometimes extensive aftercare.

Index